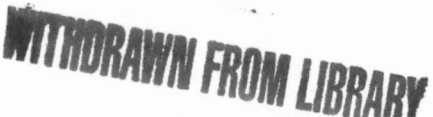

CHILD-CENTERED
PLAY THERAPY

Child-Centered Play Therapy

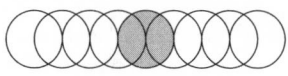

Risë VanFleet
Andrea E. Sywulak
Cynthia Caparosa Sniscak

Foreword by Louise F. Guerney

THE GUILFORD PRESS
New York   London

© 2010 The Guilford Press
A Division of Guilford Publications, Inc.
72 Spring Street, New York, NY 10012
www.guilford.com

Printed in the United States of America

This book is printed on acid-free paper.

Last digit is print number: 9   8   7   6   5   4   3   2   1

Library of Congress Cataloging-in-Publication Data
VanFleet, Risë, 1953–
    Child-centered play therapy / Risë VanFleet, Andrea E. Sywulak,
and Cynthia Caparosa Sniscak.
       p. ; cm.
    Includes bibliographical references and index.
    ISBN 978-1-60623-902-5 (hardcover: alk. paper)
    1. Play therapy.   I. Sywulak, Andrea E.   II. Sniscak, Cynthia Caparosa.
III. Title.
    [DNLM: 1. Play Therapy—methods.   2. Child.   3. Counseling.
4. Nondirective Therapy—methods.   5. Parent-Child Relations.
WS 350.4 V252c 2010]
    RJ505.P6V35 2010
    618.92′891653—dc22
                                                                        2010019293

For Bernie and Louise,
our mentors and friends,
for your pioneering work and contributions
to the fields of play therapy and family therapy,
and for the profound influence you have had on our professional
and personal development—with deep gratitude and affection

About the Authors

Risë VanFleet, PhD, is the Founder and President of the Family Enhancement and Play Therapy Center in Boiling Springs, Pennsylvania, an organization specializing in the training and supervision of child, family, and play therapy professionals. A licensed psychologist in Pennsylvania, Dr. VanFleet is also a Certified Filial Therapist-Supervisor-Instructor and a Registered Play Therapist-Supervisor. She specializes in strengthening family relationships through play. Her subspecialties include chronic medical illness in children and families; disaster mental health; child–family trauma and attachment interventions, using play therapy and Filial Therapy (FT); and canine-assisted play therapy, in which she regularly works with some of her own dogs.

Dr. VanFleet has over 35 years of clinical, supervisory, and leadership experience in a wide range of settings, and she has trained thousands of clinicians internationally. She is the author of numerous books, chapters, and articles; she is also featured on several DVD presentations. Her materials have been translated into several languages and have been used in at least 75 countries. She has been the recipient of several awards recognizing her work in the play therapy field, including the *Bernard G. and Louise F. Guerney Award for Outstanding Contributions to Practice and Training in Filial Therapy* (Association for Filial and

Relationship Enhancement Methods) and the *Play Therapy Professional Education and Training Award* (Association for Play Therapy), as well as several writing awards. She is the founder of the International Collaborative on Play Therapy and a Past President/Board Chair of the Association for Play Therapy.

Andrea E. Sywulak, PhD, is a senior partner at Sywulak and Weiss Psychological Associates, LLC, a private practice she established in 1986 in Southampton, Pennsylvania. She is licensed as a psychologist in Pennsylvania. In her private practice, she has specialized in the treatment of families with young children, utilizing FT to address the varied problems presented in childhood. She is also a Registered Play Therapist-Supervisor.

Dr. Sywulak has trained hundreds of professionals in child-centered play therapy (CCPT) and FT, and she receives regular requests to supervise other professionals in their practice of child therapy. She has given presentations on these methods and their applications at numerous local, national, and international conferences.

She also coauthored many of the early training manuals and video scripts for the Foster Parent Training Program, a statewide project in Pennsylvania in which child welfare workers were trained to teach skills derived from the principles of CCPT, to foster parents. She trained and supervised hundreds of child welfare workers as part of this project.

As a forensic psychologist dealing primarily with family issues and the effects of trauma on children, Dr. Sywulak has performed hundreds of custody evaluations, has testified as an expert witness throughout Pennsylvania, and has often been appointed as court-ordered therapist or parent coordinator. She is highly trained in trauma therapy models, including eye movement desensitization and reprocessing (EMDR) and brainspotting, which she incorporates into her CCPT and FT work.

Cynthia Caparosa Sniscak, LPC, is the President, Director, and Senior Clinician of the Beech Street Program (BSP), LLC. BSP is a private practice that offers comprehensive mental health services to children, adolescents, and families in a relaxed, playful, and family-friendly setting. Ms. Sniscak is a licensed professional counselor in Pennsylvania, a Registered Play Therapist-Supervisor, a Certified Filial Therapist-Supervisor-Instructor, and a nationally certified psychologist. She also provides canine-assisted play therapy at BSP with her cotherapist, Henry, a Labradoodle dog.

Ms. Sniscak specializes in the use of play therapy, FT, parent consultation, behavior management, and other interventions with children
and families with a wide range of problems, in particular, children with
extensive trauma and attachment problems. She works closely with
parents throughout the therapy process and coordinates her work with
school, medical, child welfare, and other mental health professionals. In
addition, Ms. Sniscak provides supervision for child and family therapists, including those using CCPT and FT. She also provides trainings
for child-related community and mental health organizations as well as
university programs. She has assisted in the development of a Pennsylvania statewide training program for law enforcement first responders
who work with abuse situations. She has been a featured speaker at
state, national, and international conferences, and has authored several
book chapters on play therapy. Ms. Sniscak was honored as the recipient of the *Family Enhancement and Play Therapy Center 2007 award for
Outstanding Contributions to Professional Training in Filial Therapy.*

Acknowledgments

We are deeply indebted to Drs. Bernard G. and Louise F. Guerney, who first introduced us to the magic of child-centered play therapy (CCPT) and Filial Therapy (FT) as systemic interventions for a wide range of child and family challenges. Their ability to translate theory into practical and effective practice is unparalleled. As this book's dedication indicates, Bernie and Louise have played a huge role in our professional development. Perhaps even more important, they epitomize the person-centered approaches that they taught us. Their acceptance, empathy, and gentle guidance are characteristics we can only attempt to emulate. Their pioneering spirit has inspired us and thousands of others around the world in the pursuit of respectful, engaging, and effective assistance for strengthening children and families.

Through the years, many child and family clients have added to our understanding of the power of CCPT. We have learned much from them, and we have appreciated the collaborative working relationships we've shared. In this manner, they have contributed to this book. Similarly, our colleagues, supervisees, trainees, and interns have helped us articulate the approach and broaden its applications, while making our professional journey a rich and rewarding one. Their impact is threaded throughout this book as well.

We are very grateful to the following people, who provided feedback on previous drafts of this volume: Harry Allen, Chris Conley, Dr. Heidi Kaduson, Claudio Mochi, Karen Pernet, Patty Scanlon, Frieda VanFleet, and Dr. Craig Weiss. Their willingness to provide their time, thoughtful suggestions, and encouragement substantially improved the quality of this book.

We also wish to acknowledge contributions of a more personal nature. Andi thanks her husband, Joe Mannino, for his unending support, encouragement, and playfulness; his patience and push helped her part of the book become a reality. Cindy is greatly appreciative of the love of family, friends, and colleagues who lent support to this undertaking with genuine encouragement and enthusiasm. Risë thanks all of her family and friends for their continual behind-the-scenes support as she took on yet another big project that minimized her time and availability.

Finally, we are grateful for the extremely supportive and encouraging environment provided to us by key people at Guilford: Rochelle Serwator, Marie Sprayberry, and Bianca Cavanaugh. Writing this book was made much easier—and much better—by their patience, knowledge, and assistance.

Foreword

As a passionate follower of Virginia M. Axline's Rogerian method of play therapy—for many more years than I care to remember!—I cannot read any type of publication on child-centered play therapy (CCPT) without experiencing a feeling of caution, until I am convinced that the author has a full grasp of CCPT and has maintained its integrity. As the authors of the present volume state, "CCPT is a more complex intervention than many people realize." Therefore, it is not uncommon for case studies in particular to be labeled in the literature as examples of CCPT when they actually bear little resemblance to the real thing. Those who have not had the opportunity to be fully educated in CCPT often personalize or otherwise modify it, to make what they believe are clinical improvements. With this book as a guide, no such errors should be made.

I had no trepidation about what I might find under the CCPT label when I agreed to write this foreword. I was sure that the authors—Risë, Andi, and Cindy, all of whom I am proud to have helped train—would create a sound and sophisticated reference. I am delighted to see what they have accomplished over the years in disseminating this model, and this book will extend their knowledge and experience to many more who wish to learn it. Of course, as should always be the case, the authors encourage readers to seek hands-on training and supervision to master the method.

For both beginners in the method and seasoned CCPT therapists, all of the content is useful, either for refreshing their memories on basics or for expanding their knowledge of additional applications or professional issues. Even when therapists have a good grasp of the basic principles and possess attitudes appropriate to the successful application of the method, there are technical dilemmas and nuances in relation to individual child therapeutic needs and responses that must be considered. Guidance is provided on a number of such points, as when children are slow to warm up for various reasons.

I was particularly pleased to see several strong chapters on extensions of CCPT practice included in the book. One of these covers another of my passions: the offshoot of CCPT known as filial therapy (FT), in which parents serve as the primary change agents conducting child-centered play sessions with their children. The training of other nonprofessionals to use nondirective child play interventions is also described.

In another chapter, the authors discuss instances in which the severity or urgency of a case is such that CCPT must be supplemented with an additional treatment. Details for combining the two treatments successfully for appropriate cases are offered; such details are rarely provided except in individual supervision. The authors make clear that this type of treatment combination is not a common practice, and they lay out guidelines for doing this discriminately. I think this discussion will be particularly helpful to therapists who are faced with a situation when progress is hampered by child, family, or social complexities.

The third is the chapter addressing the controversial subject of touch in play therapy. The authors illustrate their extensive understanding of this complex issue. Since touching and being touched are important means of communication for many children in play therapy, it cannot be ignored. Although the authors emphasize their awareness that a therapist's touch could awaken trauma in some children and could be misinterpreted by others, they believe that touch is appropriate when it is initiated by a child and when a therapist is sensitive to the child's history and perspective. They wisely caution therapists, however, that some overly wary adults may well misinterpret or misperceive touching a child. With this foreknowledge, a therapist can meet a child's needs without threatening the sensitivities of those involved.

Fourth, the authors include two chapters on dealing with adults associated with child clients. One chapter covers parents (those not conducting play sessions as in FT), as well as school personnel; the other covers social service and mental health agency personnel, together with court authorities. Because members of all these groups play an important part in making decisions for children, it is necessary that they understand what play therapy is and is not, what it can and cannot accomplish, specific benefits it can offer to children, the length of time it takes, and so forth. Specific ways to build and maintain those relationships are thoughtfully described in a way that will prove beneficial to clinicians, especially those newly faced with this bewildering world.

In sum, the book covers the basic skills of CCPT very clearly. I particularly value the emphasis on empathy, since empathy is the most powerful of the Rogerian skills. Furthermore, the authors treat broader issues of applying the method outside the playroom—in the family, school, and community—in a manner that should be of value to play therapists at all levels of experience.

I cannot close without thanking the authors for producing so fine a book that promotes the accurate understanding of this powerful method.

LOUISE F. GUERNEY, PhD, RPT-S
Professor Emerita, Pennsylvania State University
National Institute of Relationship Enhancement,
Bethesda, Maryland

Preface

Child-centered play therapy (CCPT) has been a key topic in the literature since 1947, when Virginia M. Axline, a pioneer in the method, first published her book *Play Therapy*. This was followed some years later by *Dibs: In Search of Self* (1964) and by a revised edition of *Play Therapy* (1969). Since the 1960s, many forms of play therapy—including directive, nondirective, and family-centered methods—have emerged as clinicians have recognized that play is truly the child's preferred medium of expression. Even some behaviorists now integrate play with their methods (Drewes, 2009; Ginsberg, Sywulak, & Cramer, 1984), such as when staff members of community residential facilities for developmentally disabled young adults are trained in CCPT for use with their clients. Despite the emergence, divergence, and resurgence of CCPT as a preferred method for the treatment of children with varying degrees of emotional and/or behavioral problems, the efficacy of treating children with CCPT has been established by research conducted over many years.

We three authors of this book have a total of 85 years' experience in practicing, teaching, and continually learning about CCPT. We hope to share our knowledge and experience in ways that will clarify the use of CCPT and provide detailed information about it in a user-friendly format. Today's climate of clinical practice requires clinicians to be proficient in methods that produce results. The Internet has given consumers access to vast amounts of information about therapies that can help the circumstances of their children and families. Parents are looking for proven methods to help their children when problems arise—and as the cost of services continues to rise while insurance reimbursement diminishes, they are more demanding of results.

We cannot go forward in our efforts to disseminate information about CCPT without first acknowledging the roots of our training. All three of us are deeply grateful to Drs. Bernard G. and Louise F. Guerney, the creators and pioneers of filial therapy (FT). As their graduate students and trainees, we eagerly listened to stories of the early years of their pioneering work, when the idea of putting a child in a playroom with a parent (who at that time was considered the source of the child's problem) seemed outlandish to many of their colleagues. The Guerneys took great care to ensure that parents were carefully supervised as they learned to conduct child-centered play sessions with their own children. They also conducted research to demonstrate the efficacy of their model. Careful training meant that the principles and procedures of CCPT would need to be broken down into teachable parts that could be easily understood by a layperson with no previous training. The Guerneys' clearly outlined "dos and don'ts" of CCPT have survived the years with little variation. The present book compiles all the facets of CCPT as disseminated by the Guerneys to their students over many years. Its readers will find clear and concise rules that, if followed, will enable them to practice CCPT at its most practical and highest-quality level. For those readers wishing to learn FT, proficiency in CCPT is required.

As experienced practitioners of CCPT, we have not deviated in any significant way from what we learned from the Guerneys. Our many years of practice, however, have flavored our experiences, and this volume represents our own perspectives on the practice of CCPT. Some readers may have been trained differently or may disagree with some things we have written. As practitioners and teachers of CCPT, we have often found that our own development and understanding of this method have been enhanced when clients or professionals in our training programs have challenged the rationales behind the approach. We hope that this book will open further dialogue among professionals who seek to fit CCPT more fully with their personal styles.

Because this book relates the work of Drs. Bernard and Louise Guerney, one of us (Andrea E. Sywulak) had a lunch meeting with the Guerneys during which they recounted their early experiences with CCPT and important influences on their work. Both were doctoral students in the clinical psychology program at The Pennsylvania State University in the mid-1950s. The program was influenced heavily by the work of Carl Rogers, and they were introduced to CCPT by Dr. Ila Gehman who was interested in working with children, something rare at the time. The Guerneys used Virginia Axline's 1947 book as the basis for their learning, but they were also influenced by the work of Clark Moustakas and Haim Ginott.

Because Axline's book focused on theory and did not specify methods, the Guerneys, in conjunction with Dr. Gehman, had to interpret and translate her work into the specific skills they subsequently used and taught to others, and that are detailed in the present volume. In a dynamic process, the Guerneys saw child clients, wrote reports for each session, and reviewed their work for consistency with the work of Rogers and Axline with Dr. Gehman.

We have organized this volume into five parts. Part I, "Background and Relevance," covers the importance of play, the rationale and theory of play therapy in general, and background information about CCPT. Part II, "Logistics and Techniques," covers the basic information needed to conduct CCPT, such as how to set up a playroom, what the length of sessions should be, what therapeutic skills are necessary, and how to recognize and understand children's play themes. Part III, "Parent Involvement," first discusses how to include parents (and teachers) in the CCPT process, and then describes FT as a family therapy application of CCPT. Part IV, "Practical Applications and Issues," includes ways to use CCPT with a wide range of child and family difficulties, as well as guidance in how to handle challenging behaviors and circumstances. The final part, "Research and Professional Issues," provides an overview of play therapy research and details on developing competence in the use of CCPT.

We hope that you, our readers, find this volume of interest and value. Most of all, we hope that you discover the richness of CCPT for helping children and their families make positive and lasting change.

RISË VANFLEET
ANDREA E. SYWULAK
CYNTHIA CAPAROSA SNISCAK

Contents

PART II. LOGISTICS AND TECHNIQUES

PART III. PARENT INVOLVEMENT

PART IV. PRACTICAL APPLICATIONS AND ISSUES

PART V. RESEARCH AND PROFESSIONAL ISSUES

PART I

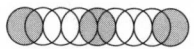

BACKGROUND
AND RELEVANCE

CHAPTER 1

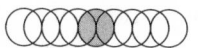

The Importance of Play

Although most people seem to recognize play when they see it, an agreed-upon scientific definition of "play" has eluded professionals from many different fields. Play seems to be enjoyable for those engaging in it, and it often involves creativity, flexibility, risk taking, curiosity, adaptability, problem solving, and "flow." Play also seems important because it occupies such a prominent place in the lives of the young. This chapter explores current and emerging knowledge about the importance of play in the lives of humans and other animals.

What Is Play?

Else (2009) has emphasized that play is a process chosen freely and directed by the players, and one that seems to be its own reward: "In summary, playing children choose the content and purpose of their actions, following their own instincts, ideas and interests, in their own way for their own reasons" (p. 11). Similarly, Clark and Miller (1998) have suggested four criteria for defining children's play: (1) It is non-literal; (2) it is done for its own reasons and not directed toward an external goal; (3) it is associated with positive feelings and is enjoyable;

3

and (4) it involves flexibility in the use of play objects as well as in the process.

While these conceptualizations of play may serve our immediate purposes, there is no universal acceptance of what play entails. The phenomenon of play has been of interest to child development experts, child mental health clinicians, biologists, comparative psychologists, historians, ethologists, anthropologists, and even dog trainers (e.g., Bekoff & Byers, 1998; Brown & Vaughan, 2009; Burghardt, 2005; Chudacoff, 2007; Elkind, 2007; Fagen, 1981; London & McConnell, 2008; Miller, 2008; Paley, 2004; Pellegrini & Smith, 2005; Sutton-Smith, 1997; Terr, 1990). Sutton-Smith (1997) identifies seven views that have been proposed through the years by professionals from several fields of study: Play is seen (1) as an adaptation that furthers development and learning; (2) as an application of strategy and skill that establishes power or hierarchy; (3) as a mechanism of optimism that offsets the negative or pessimistic side of life; (4) as a transformation from the ordinary, with its exaggerations and pretenses; (5) as an expression of one's self or identity; (6) as a means for social bonding and community building; and (7) as fun, in contrast to the world of work. The proponents of these views do not necessarily agree with each other, and may even vehemently disagree.

Burghardt (2005, pp. 45–82) provides an excellent exploration of the history, theory, and science of play, highlighting important research and proposing a five-part definition that shows promise for identifying play in human and nonhuman animals. His criteria for identifying play are as follows:

1. *Limited immediate function*. This means that the behavior is not completely focused on survival matters. Play is not serving some well-defined function that leads specifically to the player's survival. The play may have a function, but it is not immediately evident what it is. For example, the play is not designed to result in food or money acquisition, or to produce some other specific result.

2. *Endogenous component*. This means that play comes from within. It can be described as having one or more of the following attributes: It is spontaneous, voluntary, intentional, pleasurable, rewarding, and/or done for its own sake. For example, when children play, they often smile or laugh. They are motivated to continue their play activities without any adult prompting. Players of many species seem immersed in the play and convey a joyful demeanor while engaged in it.

3. *Structural or temporal difference.* This criterion posits that play behaviors differ from the "serious" forms of the behaviors in some way. Play is characterized by exaggerated expression, awkward movements, or a different sequence in the behavior pattern. Qualitative or quantitative differences distinguish it from more serious behavior. For example, in many species there are differences between play fighting and real fighting, such as different facial expressions or other signals, and the play fighting is not as rough or potentially harmful. Mouths meet more gently (dogs and other mammals inhibit their bite), and toy swords touch with at least a little more care (children inhibit the force of their blows).

4. *Repeated performance.* Play behaviors are typically repeated many times, but often with variations on the theme. For example, dogs who chase balls return for another throw over and over, often until they are exhausted. Hopscotch is a game with many repetitions of throwing the stone and hopping on the numbers on the sidewalk. Children's imaginary tea parties can involve endless pouring of water into cups, but the water may represent tea, coffee, juice, or milk throughout the play.

5. *Relaxed field.* This suggests that an animal shows little motivation to perform other behaviors when playing. The animal is more relaxed, with lower levels of stress; also, its behavior is not being influenced heavily by some other drive, such as hunger, predation, or escaping danger. Bodies seem relaxed and loose in a safe environment. If a real threat appears, play usually stops immediately. For example, two cats might enjoy a romp around the lawn together, but if the cat-unfriendly dog from next door appears, they stop playing immediately and move to a safer location. Likewise, as emphasized in this volume, children in play therapy must feel physically and emotionally safe before they truly express themselves through play.

Burghardt (2005) summarizes his five criteria into a single-sentence definition of play, with human and nonhuman animals included: "Keeping in mind the nuances underlying each word, a one-sentence definition could then read as follows: *Play is repeated, incompletely functional behavior differing from more serious versions structurally, contextually, or ontogenetically, and initiated voluntarily when the animal is in a relaxed or low-stress setting*" (p. 82). Taken together in this way, his five criteria seem to define essential features of play while ruling out alternative explanations of the behaviors.

These five criteria apply well to human play, and more specifically to children's play. Nevertheless, the discussion of "What is play?" and other questions about play will continue within, and preferably among, multidisciplinary professional groups. Burghardt's book provides an essential resource for any "serious" student of play. Furthermore, the *American Journal of Play*, which began publication of scholarly articles and research in 2008, now offers a multidisciplinary forum for the study of play.

Play and Child Development

Play is not a trivial matter. At the very least, it seems to serve important developmental purposes. Otherwise, why would the young of many species, including human children, devote so much time and exert so much energy to it? Child development specialists seem to agree that naturally occurring play is important for physical and motor development, social and emotional development, and even intellectual development (Elkind, 2007; Ginsburg, 2007; Hirsh-Pasek, Golinkoff, & Eyer, 2003; Paley, 2004; Sutton-Smith, 2008; Winerman, 2009). A report about the importance of play for children published by the American Academy of Pediatrics (Ginsburg, 2007) states: "Play allows children to use their creativity while developing their imagination, dexterity, and physical, cognitive, and emotional strength. Play is important to healthy brain development" (p. 183). Neuroscience now suggests that play helps build and strengthen neural pathways in the brain (Panksepp, 2005). Playfulness also enhances children's motivation to learn (Sutton-Smith, 2008).

Furthermore, children's free play facilitates their social development as they engage in imaginary roles and activities together, enacting family and other social scenarios through which they make decisions, solve problems, and learn from each other (Elkind, 2007; Ginsburg, 2007; Pellegrini, 2008; Perry & Branum, 2009). Both the simplicity and the safety of play allow them to negotiate and practice complex social interactions. Arguments during a children's pickup softball game ultimately help children develop social negotiation abilities, for example. Play also often has a bonding effect; people who play together often prefer to stay together. Play among peers and siblings, and with parents, helps children make stronger connections and attachments. Healthy, secure attachments permit children to explore the world on their own terms (within safe boundaries) and then return to the security of their relationships.

Changing Trends in Children's Play

With considerable concern, professionals are noting changes in the nature of children's play experiences. As play has become increasingly structured and adult-directed, the amount of time children spend in self-initiated free play has been considerably reduced. Parents and teachers, with the good intentions of providing children with optimal learning opportunities, now exert a much larger role in determining how and where and when children play. Recess periods are disappearing. Many children's lives are overscheduled, with structured activities every night and many weekends. Safe places for children's rough-and-tumble play are disappearing, as more playgrounds are paved and populated with adult-designed equipment. Rough-and-tumble play is now considered "violent" by many parents who enjoyed it as normal during their childhoods. Increasingly, adults view play primarily as a way to teach information or skills, in the hopes of improving children's academic performance and options. This trend toward more adult-determined structured play and less child-initiated free play is the result of complex societal and technological factors, and it has negative implications for children's development on many levels (Bergen, 2009; Brown & Vaughan, 2009; Chudacoff, 2007; Elkind, 2007; Ginsburg, 2007; Hirsh-Pasek et al., 2003; Honoré, 2008; Sutton-Smith, 2008; Winerman, 2009).

Sutton-Smith (2008, p. 18) poses two important questions. First, "Where does play, as a behavior, come from? Its intrinsically autonomous and fun-making character gives us good reason to believe that play has a more evolutionary character than is usually suspected." Second, "Does children's play have its own adaptive outcomes? And if so, should adults be meddling in it?" The American Academy of Pediatrics report (Ginsburg, 2007) suggests numerous ways that pediatricians and other child professionals can help educate parents about the importance of children's free and naturally occurring play for healthy development, while helping parents broaden their hopes and expectations beyond the more specific academic ones currently in vogue. It should be emphasized that parents and teachers have good intentions. They want their children to have the best opportunities, but the necessity and benefits of children's natural play tendencies are being overlooked, and consequently undermined.

It is important to remember that naturally occurring child-initiated-and-directed play is part of children's biopsychosocial makeup, and that it serves critical developmental functions as yet not fully understood. Just as one cannot accelerate the time when toddlers begin to walk and talk, it seems that many of the processes unfolding naturally within children's play cannot be rushed. Adults can provide environments that support this developmental unfolding, but they cannot anticipate it or make it happen outside its own time frame. Imposing adult ideas about play on children is likely to derail the natural processes of play that have supported the development of young humans through the ages. For this reason, it is vital for child professionals to keep abreast of theory, research, and informed dialogue in the study of children's play. On this basis, they can better educate parents, teachers, and other child professionals about the essential role of free play in many facets of healthy child development.

Assumptions about the Therapeutic Use of Play

Although the study of play yields as many questions as answers, mental health professionals who understand the importance of play in child development are increasingly adopting play-based approaches to treatment. Their aim is to provide developmentally relevant treatment in a child's own "language," that of play. The field of play therapy continues to evolve as a key approach to resolving children's psychosocial difficulties. The remainder of this volume focuses on the ways that children's play is incorporated into the treatment process, and specifically on how child-directed play is used therapeutically for a wide range of problems.

Most forms of play therapy, including child-centered play therapy (CCPT), are based on assumptions about children's play and its therapeutic value. Although most play therapists accept these assumptions, others might challenge them. Further research about the nature and purposes of play is needed to clarify its role in development and therapy. Key assumptions made by many play therapists follow.

1. Play is a drive or strong motivation that is a part of children's biological makeup. Although humans play throughout the lifespan, children do so more frequently and pervasively.

2. Play is a powerful developmental feature of childhood that contributes to child development on many dimensions. Through play, children develop motor, cognitive, affective, social, and moral capacities

and competencies. Many child development theorists have derived their ideas from observations of children's play.

3. Play expresses children's inner world—their feelings, struggles, perceptions, and wishes.

4. Play is a form of communication. Through their play, children communicate their ideas, intentions, feelings, and perceptions to their playmates, parents, and therapists.

5. Play builds social bonds. Children seek play with other children, enact social themes, and learn social behaviors and customs through play. Transgenerational play, such as when parents play with their children, builds attachment in adult–child relationships.

6. Play has a freeing effect. Play unleashes joy and excitement. It discharges distress and reduces or eliminates inhibitions.

7. Through play, children can work through and overcome their problems. The freedom of play allows them to try alternative solutions without penalty, and it provides emotional safety that enables them to explore their inner and outer worlds and apply their creativity to resolve their difficulties.

8. Play offers children an experience of power and control rarely afforded them in other situations. Children typically learn to modify their behavior in accordance with "socially accepted" norms, through the guidance of adults. In most settings, including home and school, they are expected to conform to adult rules much of the time. And in reality, the adults are the ones who have the life experience, skills, and understanding to assume control for the good of their families or organizations. In their play, however, children can take charge with less risk of harmful outcomes. Through play, they experience a sense of control while learning to manage or regulate their feelings and impulses. As they become socialized, children learn to handle power and control in adaptable ways, and play offers them a safe climate in which to do this.

9. Play occurs within many contexts. Social play in all its forms takes place in the context of relationships—with siblings, peers, parents, or therapists. Furthermore, play typically arises only when children feel safe both physically and emotionally. Play also occurs within extended social contexts, such as neighborhoods, communities, and cultures. Children play within the culture in which they are raised, and their play reflects their culture and their perceptions of their world. Even the broader sociopolitical context, such as the influence of poverty or war, can have an impact on children's play.

Albert Einstein, the Nobel Prize-winning physicist, once stated: "Imagination is more important than knowledge. For knowledge is limited to all we now know and understand, while imagination embraces the entire world, and all there ever will be to know and understand." In the interactions that parents, teachers, and child professionals have with children, it seems critical to accept and foster the children's imaginations, for their individual sakes as well as the future. Play may be the most natural and least intrusive way to accomplish this.

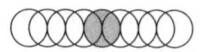

CHAPTER 2

A Brief Overview
of Play Therapy

Just as the concept of "play" does not have a single definition, neither does "play therapy." There seems to be much closer agreement among professionals, however, about what play therapy is. Consider the following four definitions.

One of us (VanFleet, 2004) has defined play therapy as "a broad field that uses children's natural inclination to play as a means of creating an emotionally safe therapeutic environment that encourages communication, relationship-building, expression, and problem resolution for the child" (p. 5).

Wilson and Ryan (2005) have described play therapy as

a means of creating intense relationship experiences between therapists and children or young people, in which play is the principal medium of communication. In common with adult therapies, the aim of these experiences is to bring about changes in an individual's primary relationships, which have been distorted or impaired during development. The aim is to bring children to a level of emotional and social functioning on par with their developmental stage, so that usual developmental progress is resumed. (pp. 3–4)

The Association for Play Therapy defines play therapy as "the systematic use of a theoretical model to establish an interpersonal process wherein trained play therapists use the therapeutic powers of play to help clients prevent or resolve psychosocial difficulties and achieve optimal growth and development" (*www.a4pt.org*, 2009).

The British Association of Play Therapists describes play therapy as

> an effective therapy that helps children modify their behaviours, clarify their self-concept and build healthy relationships. In Play Therapy, children enter into a dynamic relationship with the therapist that enables them to express, explore and make sense of their difficult and painful experiences. Play Therapy helps children find healthier ways of communicating, develop fulfilling relationships, increase resiliency and facilitate emotional literacy. (*www.bapt.info*, 2009)

Although expressed in different ways with different emphases, these definitions have much in common. They all point to *the use of systematic play interactions in the context of a therapeutic relationship in order to help children psychosocially, for the purposes of both healthier development and problem resolution.*

Although play therapy in some form has been around for a long time, many mental health professionals have misconceptions about what it actually is. For example, many therapists use toys with their child clients as a way to entice the children to talk about what is bothering them. Some therapists use more representational toys, (e.g., a family of dolls), to help their child clients focus on family issues; yet they believe that what the children talk about is more important than their play. In play therapy, whatever form it takes, *play is the therapy.* All forms of play therapy—including nondirective play therapy or CCPT, directive play therapies, and family play therapy—maintain a focus on play as a child's primary mode of expression. A *play therapist is not looking for children to be able to discuss cognitively the meaning or content of their play, but recognizes that the subconscious issues of children float to the surface through play.* Also, as the subconscious material arises, children utilize play and the environment created by the play therapist to "work through" issues that they need to address to regain emotional and social health. Although each play therapy approach is designed to help children cope with emotional difficulties, both the particular methods that are utilized and the play therapy process in general are unique to each approach. The theoretical underpinnings of each method dictate how the play therapist responds to the child and the child's play.

Types of Play Therapy

Most types of play therapy fall into one of three categories: directive or structured play therapy, nondirective play therapy or CCPT, and family play therapy. Directive play therapy involves a therapist's taking an active and leading role in the child's play, providing structure, direction, and often interpretation. Some of the more popular forms of directive play therapy include cognitive-behavioral play therapy, release play therapy, and other expressive activities that encompass some form of play. In nondirective or child-centered approaches to play therapy, the therapist is supportive but nonintrusive and allows the child self-direction. CCPT is the best-known form of (and, as noted below, is often used as a synonym for) nondirective play therapy, although some other types of play therapy are close to the nondirective end of the continuum. In family play therapy approaches, emphasis is placed on supporting the parent–child relationship and on helping parents learn skills that will build attachment and alleviate child problem behaviors and parent–child difficulties. Family play therapy can be adult-directed, as with Theraplay, or child-directed, as with Filial Therapy (FT).

Cognitive-Behavioral Play Therapy

Cognitive-behavioral play therapy uses toys and play as a means to change the thoughts and behaviors of children directly. Play materials are chosen based on the presenting problem, and are meant to meet the needs of each individual child. The underlying assumption of cognitive-behavioral play therapy is that there is a relationship among thoughts, situations, emotions, and behavior. Cognitive theory asserts that an individual's thoughts determine the person's emotional experiences and subsequent behaviors. In cognitive-behavioral play therapy, children are taught better coping skills to help them manage disturbing feelings and to decrease symptoms. Emphasis is placed on issues of control, mastery, and taking responsibility for changing one's behavior. This is accomplished through the use of playful activities initiated by the therapist with these goals in mind (Drewes, 2009; Kaduson, 2006; Knell, 1993).

Release Play Therapy

Release play therapy is a structured play therapy approach developed by David Levy (1938) and expanded by Heidi Kaduson (H. G. Kaduson, personal communication, 1995; VanFleet, Lilly, & Kaduson, 1999) for children who have experienced specific traumatic events. In release play therapy, a therapist provides an atmosphere of security and support by first allowing a child to engage in free play. Subsequently, the therapist introduces play materials needed to recreate the traumatic event, usually in miniature, so that the child may process the negative thoughts and feelings associated with the trauma in a safe environment. Levy's approach is based on a belief in the abreactive effect of play and subsequent release of the pain caused by the trauma.

Other Directive Play Therapy Approaches

Nearly every major school of psychological thought has an associated form of play therapy, such as object relations play therapy (Benedict, 2006), Adlerian play therapy (Kottman, 2002), Jungian play therapy (Allan, 2008), and the aforementioned cognitive-behavioral play therapy. O'Connor and Braverman (2009) offer a comparative approach to understanding the theoretical and practical underpinnings of most major forms of play therapy.

Storytelling, music therapy, art therapy, role playing, bibliotherapy, and other specialty therapy modalities often involve playful interactions. They can sometimes be considered forms of directive play therapy as well, because each of them puts the therapist in charge of the structure, and sometimes the direction, of the play therapy. Often these methods are used in conjunction with other forms of child therapy.

Group play therapy can be used in many settings with many ages, and can take relatively nondirective or directive forms (Kottman, Ashby, & Degraaf, 2001; Sweeney & Homeyer, 1999; VanFleet, 2009). Furthermore, some therapists use a hybrid integrating two or more forms of therapeutic intervention. Dramatic play therapy (Gallo-Lopez, 2001; Gallo-Lopez & Schaefer, 2005) combines drama therapy with play therapy. Canine-assisted play therapy (VanFleet, 2008b) integrates play

therapy with animal-assisted therapy and can be directive or nondirective in form.

Sandtray and Sandplay Therapies

In sandtray and sandplay therapies (Labovitz-Boik & Goodwin, 2000;
Lowenfeld, 1979), the therapist's office is equipped with an extensive
collection of miniature objects, sand, and water. The sand is contained
in a shallow tray with a blue bottom and sides. Children are invited
to create a world in the sandtray by moving or making patterns with
the sand and/or by placing miniature objects in the sandtray. There
are directive and relatively nondirective forms of working with sand in
play therapy. Sand-related play interventions facilitate children's use of
metaphors and symbolism, allowing them to communicate about their
world in less threatening ways.

Child-Centered Play Therapy

CCPT is a nondirective approach to helping children with emotional
and behavioral difficulties (L. F. Guerney, 2001; Landreth, 2002; Van-
Fleet, 2006a; Wilson & Ryan, 2005; Cochran, Nordling, & Cochran,
2010). A core belief in CCPT is that children have the innate capacity to resolve the problems that they are experiencing, and increase
their self-mastery, all of which results in increased competence and
self-confidence. Thus the foundation for CCPT is the belief that *the
child leads the way*. At the theoretical and philosophical center of this
approach is an appreciation for human capacity; it stresses the ability
of all clients, including children, to be self-directive in their search for
healing. This does not mean that the play therapist plays a submissive or
passive role in CCPT. In fact, the CCPT therapist's role is quite active.
The therapist unconditionally accepts and empathizes with the child
and the child's play, while following guidelines that provide safety and
structure. The therapist promotes an atmosphere that allows the child
to explore and master the self.

Sometimes a child's play in CCPT is incredibly symbolic and readily understandable by the therapist, and at other times the child's play
seems quite random and even without purpose. The following is an
example of symbolic play that occurred in a family play therapy session with an 11-year-old girl who was suffering from depression. She

was playing with her mother, who had learned FT (in which parents conduct supervised nondirective play sessions with their children; see below). During one emotional session, the girl drew a funeral scene on the blackboard, depicting her maternal grandmother's coffin at the graveside. She drew the priest performing the service, her mother, and herself, though she was the only figure with tears streaming down her face. As the mother acknowledged her daughter's drawing, her own eyes teared up. The daughter turned and asked her mother why she had never cried when Grandma died, and then fell into her mother's lap sobbing. As the mother continued to acknowledge and reflect her daughter's sadness over the loss of her grandmother and the confusion over why she herself had never cried, they held each other and cried together. When pressed to answer the daughter's question, the mother explained that she had never cried because she felt she needed to be strong for her daughter. At the end of the session, the daughter stood up, went to the blackboard, and changed the picture to depict her grandmother's coffin as buried in the ground. It was clear to both the family play therapist and the mother that the child could not symbolically bury her grandmother until she knew that she and her mother were mourning their loss together.

Ryan, age 6, was a child involved in CCPT with a therapist. His first-grade teacher had referred him because he was totally out of control in class. Although he was involved in the play therapy process for about 20 sessions, Ryan only spoke once to the play therapist: when she introduced herself and asked him his name just prior to entering the playroom for the initial session. In this first session, Ryan was somewhat aggressive as he beat up the bop bag and shot darts at various objects in the room. In the middle of the session, Ryan grabbed a box of toy soldiers and quietly began lining them up on the floor to create a battle scene. From that point onward, Ryan's play sessions consisted of setting up exactly the same battle scene with the soldiers without ever saying a word. One has to wonder what Ryan was doing and why this repetitious play was so important to him. At about the 17th session, the play therapist contacted the teacher to determine what changes, if any, were occurring in Ryan's behavior in the classroom. The teacher delightedly reported that Ryan was a totally different child; she explained that he now followed classroom rules, raised his hand instead of calling out, and was no longer acting out aggressively toward his peers or her. The teacher's only question was "What caused such a dramatic change in him?" The play therapist (who was a novice at the time) responded, "It was my magic wand." One could generate many hypotheses about what caused this dramatic change in Ryan when all he did was line up soldiers in every session. Now, with many more years of experience, the therapist understands that the powerful change agent was Ryan's self-directed play and the acceptance of self that he received during the course of his CCPT sessions.

CCPT is a fundamental approach to treating childhood problems. It is widely used by child therapists because it has clear principles and specific skills that can be broken down into teachable components. Interestingly, when the Guerneys first conceptualized FT (see below), they were convinced that CCPT was the only form of play therapy that could be taught to parents because of this teachability of the skills.

It should be noted here that in some circles, the term "child-centered play therapy" has different meanings. For many play therapists in the United Kingdom, for example, "child-centred play therapy" refers to any form of play therapy that focuses on the child's needs, whether it is non-directive or directive in nature. In the United States, "child-centered play therapy" is used synonymously with "nondirective play therapy," denoting a Rogerian/Axlinian form of play therapy in which the child selects the toys and activities and the therapist follows the child's lead. In this volume, "CCPT" is used in the latter way, interchangeably with the term "nondirective play therapy."

Theraplay

Theraplay (Jernberg & Booth, 1999; Munns, 2000, 2009; Wettig, Franke, & Fjordbak, 2006) emphasizes the relationship between the parent and child, and uses specific techniques to enhance attachment-based play and the parent–child relationship. In Theraplay there are no toys, as the therapist and the parent/caregiver are the play objects; some props or multisensory items are employed in some activities, however. Under the guidance of the therapist, the parent learns to employ engaging, nurturing, and attuned play activities that use the parent's facial expressions, physical presence, voice, rhythm, and touch as ways to elicit feelings from the child. Much of the focus in Theraplay is on nonverbal communication. An underlying assumption of Theraplay is that the parent learns to communicate with the child's right brain, which is the nonverbal part of the brain where relational information is processed.

Theraplay is considered a directive family intervention, as the adults are taking the lead and selecting or guiding the specific interactions conducted with the child.

Filial Therapy

FT (B. G. Guerney, 1964, 1969; L. F. Guerney, 1976, 1983, 1991; Sywulak, 1978, 2003; VanFleet, 2005, 2006b, 2008a; VanFleet & Guerney, 2003; VanFleet & Sniscak, 2003a, 2003b) is the premier family therapy approach for treating families with children 3–12 years old; adaptations are available for younger and older children. In FT, the parents serve as psychotherapeutic agents by learning the skills of CCPT and conducting play therapy sessions with their own children under the direction and supervision of a trained FT therapist. Developed in the early 1960s by Bernard and Louise Guerney (see the Preface), FT was conceived as a psychoeducational approach to helping families with young children. Parents learn CCPT skills, which by design strengthen the parent–child relationship. FT has all the benefits of CCPT while simultaneously improving the attunement, parenting skills, and consistency of the parents or caregivers. The goals of FT include the following: to (1) enable children to learn and understand their own feelings; (2) help children learn how to express their feelings appropriately; (3) increase trust between children and parents; (4) allow the children to work through emotional issues that underlie negative behavior; (5) increase the children's self-confidence and self-mastery; (6) increase the parents' confidence in their own parenting ability; and (7) teach parents specific skills as tools they can use for years to come. Because it is based heavily on CCPT play sessions, more information about FT is provided later in this volume (see Chapter 8).

Why Play Therapy?

Whatever forms of play therapy one practices, it is important to recognize that it is relationship-based and highly attuned to children's feelings and needs. Play is the language of children and offers therapists access to their world. Most therapists gravitate to one form of play therapy or another because of their own personality characteristics, theoretical orientation, or comfort with the skills they are employing in working with children. There is value, however, in receiving training in various forms of play therapy to expand one's knowledge base and skill sets. Despite having preferred methods for treating children, therapists sometimes need a shift in paradigm. For example, if a therapist prefers using FT but is faced with an uncooperative father and a depressed mother who does not feel comfortable conducting the play sessions, does the therapist simply give up on that child or family? Or if a therapist is working with a traumatized child who seems to have "maxed out" on the benefits of the type of play therapy used to date, shouldn't the therapist consider other methods to promote further healing and perhaps find a more suitable door into that traumatized child's world?

Today's world offers easily accessible and readily available information and training to broaden therapists' knowledge, skills, and perspectives. Dialogue about the similarities and differences in play therapy approaches can serve to expand therapists' vision and capabilities in their quest to help each child and family with whom they work.

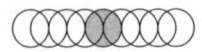

CHAPTER 3

History, Theory, Principles, and Variations of Child-Centered Play Therapy

CCPT was originally developed by Virginia M. Axline, sometime before 1947, because she recognized that "play is the child's natural medium of self-expression" (1969, p. 9). Axline had been a student of Carl Rogers, the originator and developer of client-centered therapy; she decided that if adults could talk out their problems in an atmosphere of empathy, acceptance, genuineness, congruence, safety, and self-regard, then children could play out their problems if that same atmosphere could be created in a playroom. Client-centered therapy (Rogers, 1951) is rooted in the assumption that human beings have a powerful drive not only to solve their own problems, but to strive for self-actualization. Thus there is ultimate trust in clients' own abilities to understand themselves, gain mastery over their problems, and direct their own lives in productive and emotionally healthy ways. In client-centered therapy, the therapist gives clients permission to be themselves, providing unconditional acceptance that precludes judgment or evaluation. This depth of acceptance allows clients to know who they are; to explore their unique selves; to accept themselves, and to take full responsibility for their behavior, attitudes, and emotional growth. The client-centered therapist accomplishes this by creating an atmosphere of complete acceptance, where the only commentary is an empathic listening response that acknowledges the client and his or her feelings at the deepest level of understanding.

Axline developed eight basic principles to guide the CCPT process. Although seemingly simple in nature, these guidelines provide a foundation for facilitating change and growth in child clients. Axline (1969, p. 73) outlined the eight principles as follows:

1. The therapist must develop a warm, friendly relationship with the child, in which good rapport is established as soon as possible.
2. The therapist accepts the child exactly as he is.
3. The therapist establishes a feeling of permissiveness in the relationship so that the child feels free to express his feelings completely.
4. The therapist is alert to recognize the *feelings* the child is expressing and reflects those feelings back to him in such a manner that he gains insight into his behavior.
5. The therapist maintains a deep respect for the child's ability to solve his own problems if given an opportunity to do so. The responsibility to make choices and to institute change is the child's.
6. The therapist does not attempt to direct the child's actions or conversation in any manner. The child leads the way; the therapist follows.
7. The therapist does not attempt to hurry the therapy along. It is a gradual process and is recognized as such by the therapist.
8. The therapist establishes only those limitations that are necessary to anchor the therapy to the world of reality and to make the child aware of his responsibility in the relationship.

Each of these principles is examined individually below.

Building the Relationship

Although Axline's first principle seems basic to any form of therapy, it sometimes can be particularly challenging with children. Young children, for example, tend to be mother-oriented and may have trouble separating from their mothers to enter the playroom with a therapist. Middle childhood can be fraught with issues of trust, especially if a child has felt blamed for problems in the family. To be successful in establishing the rapport necessary to do CCPT, the therapist must be highly attuned to the needs of each child and respond in an empathic way. In beginning CCPT with a very young child who may not want to separate from a parent, it may be necessary to invite the parent into the playroom with the child, and to give the parent specific directions to sit passively in the room while allowing the therapist to respond to the child. In one case where a 2-year-old had been sexually molested by a babysitter whom the mother had considered to be a friend, little Catherine could not be pried away from her mother. She was willing to go into the playroom if her mother could be with her, however. Although Catherine said nothing to the therapist for a number of sessions, the theme of the sessions revolved around such therapist responses as "You feel safe with Mommy in here," "You don't feel comfortable with me," "You keep watching me. You're not sure what you think about me," and "It's hard to play when you don't feel comfortable." Such responses finally allowed Catherine to separate physically from her mother in the playroom, and eventually to enter the playroom with the therapist alone.

It should be noted that Virginia Axline never allowed a parent to enter the playroom with a child, setting as a limit the child's entering the playroom alone. If the child did not want to go with her, Axline gave the child a choice: to wait in the waiting room alone while she spoke to the parent for an hour, or to enter the playroom with her, leaving the mother in the waiting room. Although Axline's approach to managing a child's reluctance to part from a parent is respectful of the CCPT process, we have found that parents often view it as a lack of acceptance of their children's fears. Parents may not be able to tolerate their children's distress at the very beginning of treatment, and therefore may terminate treatment. Furthermore, times and philosophies have changed in the intervening 60-plus years, and parents are included in the therapeutic process more readily today than in Axline's time.

Building rapport with a child is a process that takes time, though the time it requires varies from child to child. The relationship grows as the child begins to recognize that the CCPT therapist is consistently attuned, is nonjudgmental, allows self-direction, and consistently establishes rules that are needed to create emotional and physical safety. As the child begins to trust the process, in turn the child begins to trust him- or herself. This trust develops as the child begins to sense mastery of self and the concomitant positive regard that naturally follows.

The case of Brian offers a good example of rapport building, trust, and mastery. He lived with a single-parent father who obtained custody of Brian and Brian's twin sister when the mother chose her abusive boyfriend over her children. His mother had been given an ultimatum to get rid of the boyfriend or risk losing her children.

After spending a fair amount of time exploring the room and "feeling out" the emotional safety created by the therapist, Brian began to focus his play on the dollhouse. During many sessions, Brian created tornadoes, torrential downpours, and monsters to wipe out the contents of the house as well as the family members. He had the mother doll repeatedly jump off the roof of the house to her death. Throughout this play, Brian processed a variety of feeling states as the therapist followed his lead. Without judgment or interpretation, the therapist followed and acknowledged how scary it was to be in a house during such a violent storm, how the boy liked to have the mother jump off the roof, how unsafe it felt to be in the house, and so on. Even though it was clear that Brian was trying to gain mastery over the loss of his mother, he never identified the house as his home or the people in it as his family. Therefore, no reference was made to how his play was connected to the real turmoil he felt when his mother abandoned him, choosing an abusive boyfriend over him and his twin sister.

In this case, the therapist built rapport by unconditionally accepting Brian's use of play as metaphor. To point out the obvious connection with reality might have been intrusive or overwhelming and could have interfered with the therapeutic process.

Acceptance of the Child

At other times, children are willing but hesitant to go into the playroom with a therapist whom they have just met. Because the playroom looks enticing, and because children are used to being directed by adults, some children enter the playroom and then freeze when the therapist states: "This is a very special room. You can say or do almost anything you want in here. If there's something you can't do, I will tell you." Children who lack self-direction or confidence may stand in the center of the room and just look around. Others may stand there and cry. Because it is painful for therapists to see children struggle, a basic instinct is to comfort such a child or help the child "get started" by introducing some toy or activity. In CCPT, it is not the job of the therapist to "take care" of the child, but rather to accept that child exactly where he or she is. Appropriate empathic responses in such situations might include "You're nervous about being in here with me," "It's hard to get comfortable when you're with someone that you don't know," "You're afraid you'll do the wrong thing," or "You're upset at being someplace new and don't know what to do." It is important to remember that true acceptance is tuning in to the feelings of the child exactly as that child is in the moment.

Although Axline (1969) recommended that therapists remain silent if children were silent and should busy themselves with notes or doodling until the children revealed some type of feeling, we recognize that long silences can be emotionally threatening to some children. Silence is often interpreted as disapproval. For example, adults often "give the silent treatment" when children (or other adults, for that matter) are doing something of which they disapprove. Although Axline took notes during sessions, this is rarely done by current CCPT therapists. One cannot take notes and be fully child-centered at the same time. We believe that any activity that pulls a CCPT therapist's total attention away from a child conveys something negative to the child, such as lack of interest or ignoring "inappropriate" behavior. Continually conveying acceptance, through comments made about what the play therapist is observing about the child, builds the atmosphere of genuine interest and acceptance from the first few moments the child and therapist enter the playroom and throughout the session.

One question often asked by novice play therapists is whether acceptance is misinterpreted by children as agreement with the children or approval of the children's behavior. It is important to remember that aside from setting the limits required for physical and emotional safety, a therapist makes no judgment about a child's play. An assumption of CCPT is that children are doing exactly what they need to do at any given time in order to work on their own problems. For example, if a child decides to spill water over some of the toys and on the carpet, the CCPT therapist would respond by saying something such as "You're having fun pouring the water on those things," or "Sometimes it's fun to get things wet." If the child looks for a reaction from the therapist, the therapist might say, "You're wondering what I think about your spilling the water." If the child insists on knowing what the therapist's reaction is, the CCPT therapist simply responds, "You really want to know what I think. Remember, you can do just about anything you want to in the special room." (It should be noted that in the case of spilling water, therapists can manage the amount of dampness in the playroom by limiting the amount of water available. For example, the therapist might include just 1 or 2 cups of water in a small bottle. This allows children to engage in spilling play without soaking the playroom for subsequent clients.)

Establishing a Sense of Permissiveness

Permissiveness is established when the CCPT therapist uses an accepting tone, maintains genuine interest in the child's play with nonjudgmental facial expressions, and behaves in a nonjudgmental and nondirective manner. Early in treatment, children in CCPT explore the room and are mindful of the therapist's responses or actions, which can either convey permissiveness or not. Children are so attuned to the way adults relate to them that even simple gestures can limit a child's sense of permissiveness in the playroom. For example, if the child overfills a cup with water, the water then runs off the edge of the play sink, and the therapist takes a sponge to prevent the rug from getting wet, the therapist has conveyed through that one action a lack of permissiveness.

Permissiveness in CCPT does not mean that a child is free to do anything at all; as we describe later, there are rules that are enforced at appropriate times in a therapeutic manner. The permissiveness described here refers to the therapist's giving children permission to express whatever they are thinking and feeling at the moment in the playroom.

Permissiveness in the relationship between a child and a play therapist is part and parcel of every play therapy encounter. It requires consistency on the part of the therapist to maintain permissiveness by avoiding any direction for the child, any introduction of topics, or any probing questions, no matter how "innocent" they may seem. Therapists may innocently or unwittingly cross these boundaries, but by doing so, they are putting their own imprint on therapy sessions rather than allowing children to lead the way. Just as negative judgment is inappropriate when one is trying to create a permissive atmosphere, so too is approval, praise, or encouragement. All judgment, be it positive or negative, sends a message to a child about the therapist's expectations with regard to the child's play. For example, if a child is throwing bean bags at the bean bag board, continues to fail to get a bean bag through one of the holes, and seems frustrated, it would be inappropriate to say, "You're trying hard. You can do it." The subtle message sent by the play therapist is that the child should continue the activity until he or she succeeds. This may cause the child to feel bad if he or she doesn't succeed, because the therapist might be disappointed. Instead, a better response would be "You're really frustrated! It's hard to get those bean bags through the holes."

The foundation of a healthy relationship in CCPT is built on the rapport that is established through the play therapist's consistent attitudes of acceptance and permissiveness. The child learns to trust and have confidence in the therapist, in a manner that allows the child to feel safe enough to begin revealing deep feelings. With some children, this trust develops relatively quickly. For example, Joey was a severely abused child who lived with foster parents. In his first session, Joey covered his face with two masks that were in the playroom. He also told the play therapist that he had to wear the masks because the boy who was under them was so ugly and dirty that the therapist wouldn't like him. Because the play therapist maintained a posture of acceptance and permissiveness, Joey slowly began to remove each mask until his face was uncovered. By the end of the session, Joey felt safe enough to fill a baby bottle with water, and to cuddle up like a baby on the therapist's lap as he cooed and sucked the bottle. Although this is not the most typical first play session with an emotionally disturbed child, it serves to emphasize the power of acceptance and permissiveness in creating the safety a child needs to explore vulnerable feelings. With many children with emotional and behavioral problems, this is a much slower process, because the children's prior experience with adults is that they cannot express themselves and feel safe. All that is required of the therapist is to be empathic, be patient, and to trust the CCPT process—that is, to allow the child's issues to unfold at a pace the child is able to manage. The payoff is that children will develop mastery over their thoughts, feelings, and behavior.

Empathic Recognition and Reflection of Feelings

The very essence of the CCPT process is the therapist's use of "empathic listening" or "reflective listening." It is through the proper use of this skill that the CCPT therapist is able to create the atmosphere in the playroom that establishes acceptance, permissiveness, and the basis for a secure relationship with the child. Empathic listening is a skill of attunement, beginning with the recognition of feelings and culminating in a response that actively conveys the identified feelings in an accepting and nonjudgmental manner to the child. It is not meant to be a mechanical repetition of what the child says, nor is it an ana-lytical interpretation of the child's words or play. At times an empathic response may be a simple description of what the child is doing, but whenever possible, the best responses include the use of feeling words that are in tune with the child's play. For example, if a young child pours a pitcher full of water into the sink and starts splashing the water with his or her hands while giggling, an acceptable empathic listen-ing response would be "You're splashing in the water." An even bet-ter response would be "You're really enjoying yourself. It's fun to splash in that water." An interpretive response, which is inappropriate in the CCPT approach, would be "You like splashing in the water because you aren't allowed to do that outside of here."

Empathic or reflective listening is a therapeutic skill that appears easy, but some child therapists have a difficult time with it. Empathy requires therapists to "get out of their own heads and into children's heads." Children are usually transparent, and by listening to their vocal inflections, looking at their faces, and studying their body language, one can usually determine what they are thinking and feeling. Empathic listening involves the therapist's stating what is observed in this way. The therapist is attuned to what the child is saying and doing, and comments on it while recognizing the emotions the child is explicitly or implicitly conveying.

Essentially, the play therapist's use of empathic listening sets the tone for each CCPT session. Of all the skills used in the playroom, empathic listening comprises the majority of comments made by the CCPT therapist. These responses, however, are not meant to be a running commentary on every detail of a child's play; rather, they are thoughtful, accepting responses indicating that the therapist is attuned to and interested in the child's play. To accomplish this, the CCPT therapist uses the skill of empathic listening in a gentle, nonintrusive, almost rhythmic manner, but with an inflection that lets the child know the therapist understands how he or she is feeling. Once the child trusts the therapist and the process of CCPT, the therapist may respond less frequently, though this is generally in later stages of the therapy. As stated earlier, long periods of silence should be avoided, so that they do not undermine the therapist's nonjudgmental stance. Furthermore, when therapists try to "pick and choose" the timing of their empathic responses, it is easy for their own biases to exert an influence. For exam-ple, it is common for new CCPT therapists to readily reflect feelings such as excitement or enjoyment, while remaining silent about feelings of sadness or anger. In CCPT, it is important for a therapist to accept *all* of a child's feelings, and this is accomplished through the effective use of empathic listening.

Axline (1969) wrote about not reflecting direct questions from the child, to avoid bogging down the play therapy process during the exploration phase of CCPT. In fact, we have found the exact opposite to be true. In other words, when therapists reflect direct questions with "You're wondering what that is," or similar comments, children quickly learn to trust their own ideas and to express their own feelings more directly. We all must remember that as adults, we question children all the time. As a consequence, children learn to ask questions as a way to communicate with others. Yet questions are often inadequate expressions of feelings. For example, if a child is rushing to complete some activity, nervously looks at the clock, and asks, "How much time do we have left?", the most appropriate empathic listening response is not "Two minutes," but rather "You're worried that you're not going to have enough time to finish that." Interestingly, the child usually feels satisfied knowing that the therapist understands the child's dilemma. Also, with very young children, the reflection of questions such as "What is this?" often leads to some interesting and creative play when the therapist answers, "You're wondering what that is," or "You're trying to figure out what that is; you're not sure."

In a play session 3-year-old Helena held up various toys and asked repeatedly, "What is this?" When the therapist continued to respond, "You're wondering what that is," Helena relied on herself and came up with some very creative ideas. For example, when she asked about several darts that she held in her hand, and the therapist replied, "You're wondering what those are," Helena responded by handing the darts to the therapist and stating, "Here, they're flowers." Then when she asked what the dart gun was and heard from the therapist, "You're trying to figure that out," Helena turned the gun upside down, looked through the part where the trigger was, and said, "Smile! It's a camera, and I'm going to take your picture."

Helena's responses raise the important question of how much creativity adults actually squelch in children. Armed with preconceived notions from the adult perspective, parents, teachers, and even therapists probably provide too many answers or too much direction. In CCPT, empathic listening allows therapists to tune in to children's world of play and respond in ways that let children know the therapists are with them and interested in their play and their ideas.

Some of the most difficult play sessions occur with children who do not speak during the session and are undemonstrative in their actions and gestures. Such was the case with Jack, an 11-year-old boy, whose parents had recently separated and were in the middle of an acrimonious divorce. When Jack entered the playroom for the first time, he lay across the bop bag and just stared at the play therapist. When the play therapist reflected, "You're not sure what to do in here," Jack responded, "Nope." As Jack continued to lie on the bop bag and roll around a bit, the play therapist reflected, "You seem bored. It's hard to figure out what to do in here." Jack responded, "Yep." Through most of this first session, Jack continued to lie on the bop bag, look longingly at the play therapist, or casually look around the room. The play therapist continued to reflect his actions and, whenever possible, his feelings. Empathic listening comments included statements such as "You're looking at something over there," "You're not sure what you want to play with," "It's hard getting started when you're someplace new," or "You're looking at me and wondering what you're supposed to do in here." Again, Jack responded in the affirmative to all the reflective commentary, but seemed immobilized. To a seasoned CCPT therapist, however, such unwillingness to play and lack of expression are not problematic. They simply require the play therapist to stay attuned to the child and create an atmosphere of acceptance and permissiveness until the child is ready.

By the second session, Jack continued his reluctance to play or speak until the last 5 minutes of the session. At that point, with a forlorn look on his face, Jack simply asked the play therapist whether she knew that his parents had separated. The play therapist acknowledged that she knew this and reflected back, "You wanted to make sure I knew that. You seem pretty sad about it." And Jack responded, "Yep." During the third session, Jack became more animated and started to play in an aggressive (though still controlled) way with the bop bag and dart guns. The father reported to the play therapist that his son had always been uncomfortable with expressing feelings, but was extremely sensitive. Children like Jack will need to make sure that the playroom is a safe enough place to reveal themselves before they can do so.

Years ago, while teaching a class on the value of empathic listening, Bernard Guerney related a story about a session Carl Rogers held with an adolescent client. Rogers had seen the teenager in individual client-centered therapy for about a year. Rogers reported that the boy never spoke during the entire time, but sat there looking at him or staring out the window. Reportedly, Rogers continued to accept his silence and would make some reflective comments when he thought it was appropriate. In a final session, the young man reported to Rogers that he was feeling much better and ready to end therapy. Rogers, being curious as to what helped the boy, asked him what helped make the change. The young man replied that Rogers was the first person to accept him totally as he was, never forcing him to speak, but being totally present with him. What an illustration of the power of acceptance and attunement!

Respecting the Child's Ability to Solve Problems

At the core of client-centered therapy is the belief that, given the appropriate atmosphere, all people are capable of solving their own problems. In CCPT, there is absolute belief in children's ability to solve their own problems through play, given an appropriate play therapy atmosphere. In CCPT, children learn that they are completely responsible for themselves and their behavior.

For example, Robbie, a 7-year-old boy who was referred because of problems with self-control, soon learned the power of self-responsibility. Although Robbie was thrilled upon entering the playroom, his exuberance and lack of self-control soon led to his shooting the therapist with the darts three times—thus ending the play session within minutes of its start, in accordance with the limit-setting skill of CCPT (see Chapter 5). With each successive session, Robbie extended his playtime by some minutes, but still could not refrain from breaking the limit by shooting the therapist three times. (It should be noted that the remainder of the "therapy time" involved having Robbie sit in the waiting room as the play therapist spoke to his mother about Robbie's self-control issues and why it was important to end each session after a rule was broken for the third time.) After five or six sessions like this, Robbie began to recognize that he ultimately had control over being able to spend the entire time in the playroom; he began choosing to shoot the dart gun everywhere except at the therapist, no longer necessitating the limit setting.

During his subsequent play therapy sessions, Robbie expressed much anger and frustration as he shot the dart gun, punched the bop bag with as much force as he could muster, spilled water all around the room, and threw various toys about the room without ever once hitting the therapist with anything. Then one day, Robbie settled into building with bristle blocks until the 1-minute warning, when Robbie promptly shot the therapist with a dart, smiled at the therapist, and walked out of the playroom; he thereby ended the session a few moments earlier, but did so under his own control. The therapist responded by stating, "You enjoyed shooting me again. It's important to you to be in charge of ending the session." Following that session, Robbie's play focused on issues of self-mastery—being able to obtain a high score when shooting darts at the target, getting all six bean bags through the holes in the bean bag board without missing, and so on. With each passing session, his mother talked to the therapist about all the positive changes she was seeing in Robbie at home and in school. Although it had been difficult for Robbie's mother to understand the rationale for ending the first five play sessions after only a few minutes, she now came to understand the value of the therapist's respect for Robbie's ability to work through and solve his own problems.

Because of the CCPT therapist's deep respect for children's ability to solve their own problems, any way a child chooses to play or not to play is considered what the child needs to do in order to achieve mastery of self and the play environment. It does not matter if the child is overly dependent, fearful, boisterous, outspoken, anxious, aggressive, or withdrawn. The CCPT therapist has confidence in all children's ability to figure out what they need to resolve their emotional and behavioral difficulties and to learn to trust and accept themselves. As they play within this trusting, permissive, and accepting atmosphere, children come to sense the play therapist's trust in them. This in turn allows children to develop their own sense of trust in self, self-acceptance, and self-responsibility. Therefore, when a child struggles to load a dart gun, make a basket with a Nerf basketball, untie a knot in a jump rope, or the like, the CCPT therapist feels comfortable not jumping up to help or not instructing, but simply responding to the frustration or determination the child is feeling.

In fact, if children clearly ask for help, CCPT therapists offer assistance, but do so in the least intrusive manner possible. For example, a therapist waits for a child to hand the dart gun to him or her to load it. If the child continues to struggle to load the dart gun and halfheartedly asks, the therapist waits and reflects back to the child, "You're frustrated," "That's hard to do," or "You're really trying hard to do that by yourself." Most of the time, with this kind of acceptance and nonintrusiveness on the part of the play therapist, children are ultimately successful in accomplishing the task for which they initially thought they needed the therapist's help. The result is that the children are delighted as they experience mastery. The play therapist then simply acknowledges this: "You are really proud of yourself for figuring that out." On the other hand, but similarly, if a child has great difficulty asking for help, the time often comes in play sessions when he or she asks for the therapist's assistance. To deny the child's need and the child's request might be to deny growth in this area. The therapist therefore follows the child's lead, reflects the need ("You're having trouble and want me to show you how to do that"), and then assists as the child has asked. As always, the therapist respects the child's ability to determine what is needed; in this case, it would be to reach out to others rather than always going it alone.

Again, just as children ask questions for which they are not really looking for answers, they often ask for help from an adult when they really don't want or need it. In CCPT, the unwavering commitment of the play therapist to respecting children's ability to solve their own problems leads to mastery of self, responsibility for self, and ultimately enhanced self-esteem as children learn that they are capable of solving their own problems. We must ask ourselves, if tempted to help a frustrated child who has not requested help, how the child will learn to cope with frustration (or any feelings, for that matter) if adults are there to solve all his or her problems. Also, if, as adults, we take the responsibility for solving all the child's problems, aren't we in fact "putting little dents" in the child's self-esteem by inadvertently sending a message about dependence and helplessness ("You can't do that, so I must do it for you")?

Letting the Child Lead the Way

Another key element of CCPT is the inherently nondirective nature of the therapy. It is totally up to the child—not the play therapist—to decide whether or not to play, whether or not to talk, and what the play or talk is going to be. In other words, while being attuned to the child, the CCPT therapist waits patiently to follow as the child leads the way. One of the best ways to understand this concept is to examine the "don'ts" of CCPT. These include no directing, no judgments, no teaching, no suggestions, no praise, no criticism, no interpretation, and no questions.

Directing the child would be an obvious deviation from the nondirective stance, though it can be tempting for a novice play therapist to help out a little. For example, if the child's hands are wet from playing in the water and there are no paper towels left, the play therapist might be tempted to say, "You can use the baby blanket to dry your hands." A correct response would be "You don't like your hands to be wet. You're not sure how to dry them off." In CCPT, it is up to the child to determine the solution to this dilemma.

Judgments can inadvertently occur when the novice play therapist makes a point of laying out toys in a conspicuous manner, which could cause the child to think that those toys are the ones he or she should play with. For example, if the play therapist believes the child is having trouble expressing anger, it could be tempting to place all the aggression toys (see Chapter 4) in the center of the room, to encourage aggressive play in an effort to elicit angry feelings from the child. Children are extremely sensitive to adult attitudes, even when these are unspoken, and may feel pushed to do something they are not ready to do to please an adult. When therapists make judgments about what they think children need in play therapy, they are negating their respect for children's ability to do what they need to solve their own problems.

Because children are in the process of learning about many things, they often seem inadequate in their abilities. As adults, it is easy to forget that learning is a process, and that children have an innate drive to learn and master their environment and themselves. Therefore, there is a temptation to teach, especially when adults see an opportunity in children's play to help them learn something that the adults deem important. An example is when a child plays the teacher role at the blackboard in the playroom and either spells a word wrong or adds two numbers incorrectly. The child may look at the word or numbers and seem confused. An appropriate reflective comment would be "You look confused. You're not sure if you did that right." Sometimes this response results in the child's correcting the mistake him- or herself. At other times, the child may ask the therapist if the word or math is correct. When asked directly, the CCPT therapist might say first, "You're wondering if you did that right," and then (if pushed by the child to answer), "You want me to tell you if you did it correctly." When, and only when, the child affirms that he or she wants correction does the play therapist say, "No, that isn't quite right." If asked for the correct answer, the therapist would first say, "You want me to help and tell you the right answer." When the child affirms this, the play therapist can then tell the child the correct answer. In some cases, the child simply proceeds with the activity and does not notice the mistake. If that is the case, an appropriate response might be "You like being the teacher. You want to write more words [do more problems]."

Sometimes children will lead therapists to think that they want input in making decisions about their play, perhaps by asking something like "What do you think I should play with?" The novice play therapist might think that the child desires some direction. In our own experience, however, children sometimes do this in the early stages of play therapy because they don't feel that comfortable with the self-direction offered in the CCPT setting. It is important to remember that children are quite used to adults' taking the lead outside play therapy sessions, and may not quite trust the permissive atmosphere that the therapist has established. An appropriate response might be "You're wondering what I think you should do," or "You're not sure what is okay to do in here." If the child responds in the affirmative, the next best response is "Remember you can do almost anything you want to in here." If the child continues to push the issue, the therapist might reflect, "You really want me to help you make the decision about what to do." If the child responds affirmatively, it is okay to say, "Well, you could choose to play with the bean bags, the dart guns, or the watercolors, or anything else." In this way, the therapist avoids the direct suggestion of an activity, but informs the child of some possible choices. Occasionally a child strongly pushes the therapist to decide by saying something like "I like the bean bags or the checkers, but I want you to choose." A CCPT therapist first reflects, "You want my help in making the decision about what to play with," or "You want me to be happy." If the child responds affirmatively and just waits for an answer, it is then okay for the therapist to make a choice. After the therapist makes such a choice, however, it is common for children to choose something totally different from or even opposite to the therapist's selection. The therapist would follow this up with an empathic response such as "You don't like my suggestion. You would rather play . . ." Although this may seem like an arduous process, the benefit to the children can be enormous. For one thing, children learn that it really is up to them to take the lead, and that the play therapist will accept their choices when they do. Also, children learn to trust the permissive atmosphere of the playroom, so that they feel free to express themselves in whatever way is most meaningful to them.

Praise and criticism are also judgments and therefore play no part in the CCPT session. Even when children seem to be looking to therapists for some type of evaluation, it is vital to remember that therapists' evaluations of them are insignificant, in that it really does not matter what therapists think or believe in the CCPT setting. Instead, being a CCPT therapist means mirroring the feelings children reveal. For example, the child paints a picture, holds it up, and asks, "Do you like this?" It order to make an appropriate response, the CCPT therapist must be attuned to the nuances in the child's tone or facial expression. Depending on what the therapist observes, he or she might say, "You're proud of your picture and want to know what I think," or "You seem disappointed in your picture, and you're not sure if I will like it." Often the simple acknowledgment of the child's feeling is sufficient and satisfying for the child, and no further commentary is required. If the child persists in requesting the therapist's evaluation, the CCPT therapist first reflects the child's desire for the opinion and offers a gentle though positively toned appraisal, such as "I like it too," or "I like all the colors you used." (Here the therapist is making a judgment only because the child has pushed for it.) The therapist might underscore the child's lead role in the session by adding, "But in here, it's what you think that counts." It is important to remember that all judgment is reserved until the play therapist has exhausted every opportunity to reflect and acknowledge the child's feelings and intent for wanting the judgment. Very often, a child keeps pushing for an answer to a question because the play therapist has not yet captured the true meaning of what the child is trying to convey. What the therapist must do is try to see the deepest level of feelings or intentions in the child's play and make sure that the reflections capture them. The child needs to feel that the therapist understands the core or the essence of the message.

Interpretation or analysis plays no role in CCPT, as these types of responses assume that a play therapist knows more about what a child needs to heal than the child does. When a play therapist makes an interpretive comment, the attunement with the child diminishes. The more interpretive the comments made by the play therapist, the less control the child has over the direction of the play, as the play becomes what it means to the therapist and not to the child. Suppose the therapist knows from a parent's report that the child has a history of cruelty to animals. Although the child's play in the therapy room has been generally aggressive, the child likes to cuddle and care for a stuffed teddy bear. It would be interpretive to say, "You need to take care of that bear because you feel so guilty about hurting real animals." A more appropriate response from a CCPT therapist would be "It feels good to cuddle that bear. You enjoy taking care of it." When one is tempted to assign intent or psychological meaning to the child's play, or to use the word "because" in a reflective response, it is likely that the response is an interpretive one and should be avoided.

Questions are avoided in CCPT because they are considered to be directive and can cause children to change the nature or direction of their play. Although attorneys use questions to get information, many times their intent is to make witnesses defensive and confused. This is often the case if a play therapist asks questions. It is very easy for a child to misperceive the intent of these questions. It may cause the child to think, "What does the therapist want from me?" or "What is the 'right' answer?" Also, the child may think that he or she is doing something wrong. Questions make people, including children, feel defensive and put on the spot. CCPT therapists are not interested in helping children gain insight by understanding the meaning of their play; therefore, any "Why?" question serves no purpose. Most adults have been in situations where they ask children why they did something (e.g., hit a sibling), only to have the children shrug their shoulders and say, "I don't know." In fact, children often have no idea why they did what they did, so "I don't know" is an honest answer. Children are only beginning the process of understanding themselves and their behavior. Much of children's behavior is determined by how they are feeling; yet they have not mastered the language of feelings, so they will often act out their anger, frustration, disappointment, hurt, and so on.

In CCPT, therapists strive to help children learn the language of feelings by mirroring or reflecting back to them what the therapists believe they are feeling. Some novice play therapists worry that if they state a feeling word about children's indirect expressions, instead of asking children directly about their feelings, they are putting the idea into the children's heads. In fact, the opposite seems to be true. If a CCPT therapist mistakenly identifies the wrong feeling word, children typically and freely correct the therapist and disagree with the feeling word used. For example, if a therapist states, "You are proud of your picture," and the child is not, the child will say, "No, I'm not." In this situation, the best thing to do is to accept the child's rejection of the feeling by stating, "You're not proud of your picture, and you want me to know that." Sometimes a child disagrees with the reflection of a feeling, especially anger, if the child is not ready to disclose that particular feeling to the play therapist. In such situations, questioning whether the child feels anger would only serve to make the child more defensive about his or her anger, and perhaps more inclined to bury the angry feelings. For example, if a child is angrily beating up the bop bag, and the therapist reflects, "You are angry and really letting that guy have it," and the child says, "No, I'm not. I just like punching him," the best CCPT response is "You want me to know you're not angry. You are just having fun punching him really hard."

Treating Play Therapy as a Gradual Process That Cannot Be Hurried

More than ever, children are growing up in a world where the pace of life is in high gear. Children learn things in third grade that used to be taught in junior high school. Their parents run them from one organized activity to another each day after school; for many such children, it is difficult to set up therapy appointments that do not conflict with some activity. Computers give children access to information that only adults were privy to before. Children are taught by high-striving parents that "success" means having a $100 haircut, designer clothes, and all the latest technology. Because children have learned to become so enthralled with contraptions that provide them with entertainment, it can be a challenge for a play therapist to go into a toy store and find simple, basic toys that are appropriate for play therapy. Parents are impatient with children as they try to master some basic things, such as learning to button their own coats, tie their own shoes, or struggle through math problems. Many parents admit that they do way too much for their children because they don't have time to wait for the children to do it themselves. As a result, children feel entitled, yet dependent; boastful, yet insecure; idealized, yet inept.

Childhood is actually a very brief period of every person's life. It spans just 18 years. It is said that more learning occurs during the first 5 years of a child's life than in the remainder of that child's lifetime. Because the world is a very big and complex place, children have lots of information to learn, master, and integrate in order to become the persons they will be. At a very basic level, however, a child is learning about him- or herself and how to be and relate in the world. Learning about and mastering the self is the most important facet of learning in childhood. It establishes the child's personality and how that child will relate to others in this complex world. It is a process that cannot be hurried, as the child needs time, space, and acceptance to complete this process in a healthy fashion.

CCPT gives children all the time they need to learn about themselves and to practice mastery. Play therapists have confidence in children's ability to get to where they need to be, and they are patient with the children's process—whatever it may be and however long it may take. Yet it is amazing how much learning occurs in a relatively short period of time in a playroom where a child's self is the focus. As CCPT therapists, we have learned to appreciate and enjoy the atmosphere of the playroom. In many ways, it relieves therapists of the pressures many feel "to make things happen" and to solve children's problems as they have been presented by the parents. CCPT therapists know that with attunement, acceptance, patience, and good limits, each child will set out on a course of self-improvement and self-actualization. Therapists convey to children that they are not in a hurry, because the therapists patiently follow the children's lead and do not push them in any way. The therapists do not rush in to solve their dilemmas, nor do the therapists have any expectation of what the children must accomplish during the therapy hour. CCPT therapists allow children to be who they are and enjoy their relationships with those children as the children permit. It is truly a freeing experience for children and therapists alike.

The Importance of Limits

The limits that are established in CCPT are very few, but are of utmost importance. Limits help children know that the play therapist will maintain an atmosphere of safety in the playroom, especially when the children feel out of control of their own feelings. When adults do not establish good limits, children feel anxious and insecure. Many children will push adults to establish limits by escalating their negative behavior. Because children rely on adults for the safety limits they provide, children cannot build rapport with or maintain respect for a play therapist who does not maintain a clear and consistent limit structure.

One clear example of the value of limits in play therapy occurred in an FT play session where Audrey, a 6-year-old who was referred because she was selectively mute, was playing with her father. Although he was quite intelligent and clearly understood the reasons for setting limits, Audrey's father struggled to do this with her both at home and in the play sessions. In one session, Audrey needed to test the safety of the playroom, so she began to hit her father, first with Nerf toys and then with the bop bag. Her behavior then escalated to throwing wooden toy furniture at him, in a desperate effort to get him to stop her. The father continued to be very accepting and simply could not bring himself to state the limit that he was not to be hit with anything. The FT therapist knew that he would have to be pushed to do so, and accomplished this by stating over the office's loudspeaker system to the father: "Remember the rule is you can't be hit with anything. Tell her that!" The father was so surprised at the FT therapist's intervention that he blurted the rule out to Audrey. Upon hearing this from her father, Audrey stopped hitting him with anything; she then exploded into angry and aggressive play directed at everything in the room except her father. The next day, Audrey began to speak "yes" and "no" answers in school. In a short time, she was talking normally to her teacher and peers. Her father immediately understood that when he finally set the limit about being hit, Audrey was free to express the anger she had bottled up inside of her, as the limit made it safe for her to do that. Audrey's father learned a valuable lesson that he was now able to generalize to their home life. Once he established limits for Audrey in the playroom and at home, Audrey was free to express herself without having to worry that her anger could get so far out of control that she might hurt someone.

Children learn self-control and appropriate feeling expression through the use of good limits and consequences. The application of limits and consequences in a three-step process (described in detail in Chapter 5) allows children to learn that they are responsible for their own behavior, and that they have a choice as to whether or not to continue to break a rule. Because children enjoy and look forward to their play therapy sessions, they soon learn that the risk of no self-control leads to the termination of a session. Once children learn that they can have control over themselves and that appropriate expression of feelings leads to release of pent-up emotions and anxiety, the CCPT sessions become a haven of safety to do the work they need to do. As a child's "work" is accomplished in CCPT, the child soon learns to self-regulate, and then generalizes what he or she learns in the therapy room to the outside world.

Six-year-old Colin was referred for treatment because his behavior was out of control both in school and at home. His mother reported that Colin's father had an active alcohol problem and was physically abusive. She felt trapped in the marriage, however, because her family refused to help her and the children leave this horrible situation. The mother was clinically depressed and not responding to medication. She felt compelled to get Colin help, because the school complained to her every day about his behavior. She was not willing to get help for herself, but dutifully brought Colin to his play therapy session each week. Two sessions with Colin were memorable with regard to his response to limit setting.

In the first session, Colin angrily tore the playroom apart. Toys went flying everywhere. Furniture was turned up on end. He spilled the whole pitcher of water all over the toys and the floor. Then Colin stood in the center of the mess, realizing that the mess made it difficult to play. He found a piece of paper and the watercolors and stated, "I'm gonna paint!" Much to his dismay, the watercolors were dry, and he had already emptied the pitcher of water all over the playroom. The interchange then went as follows:

COLIN: I need to go get more water so I can paint. (*Tucks the pitcher under his arm and is about to leave the playroom.*)

THERAPIST: Colin, remember there are some rules. One of them is that you can't leave the playroom, except to go to the bathroom. Otherwise, the play session will be over.

COLIN: (*Has a bright idea.*) I have to go to the bathroom. (*Is still holding the pitcher tucked under his arm.*)

THERAPIST: Colin, remember there are some rules. One other rule is that you can't leave the playroom with any of the toys. [Exceptions are only made for pictures children draw or objects they create out of clay.]

COLIN: Okay, I'll just go to the bathroom. (*Returns within minutes, holding two little cups of water he has gotten from the bathroom cup dispenser.*)

THERAPIST: Colin, remember there are some rules. Another rule is that you can't bring anything into the special room. (*Frustrated, Colin goes back to the bathroom, dumps the cups of water into the sink, and throws out the cups.*)

COLIN: I really want to paint. (*Looks around the room, trying to figure out how to accomplish this.*)

THERAPIST: You're disappointed that you don't have water to paint. You're trying to figure out what to do about this.

COLIN: (*Eyes light up as he looks in the mess for a little kitchen cup.*) I know what I'm going to do.

THERAPIST: You're proud that you figured out a way to handle your problem.

Colin proceeded to head toward a puddle of water on the rug, scooped what water he could from it with his hands, and sprinkled it into the little cup. Having retrieved only a few drops of water, Colin tried in vain to paint a picture. Frustrated again, Colin threw down the paintbrush and walked out of the room. The therapist responded, "Colin, you're really frustrated that you can't paint, so you want to end the session. Remember, if you leave, the play session is over for today."

The following session, Colin happily entered the playroom. The therapist said, "You seem really happy today. You're anxious to get started." Colin then took a small cup from the play kitchen, filled it with water, safely placed it on the windowsill, and looked proudly at the play therapist. "You seem proud that you figured something out. You want to save that water for something special." With that, Colin promptly made a mess of the room just as he had done in the previous session. Then he picked up a piece of paper, fetched the watercolors, and retrieved the little cup of water he had saved on the windowsill. The therapist responded, "You had fun making a big mess. You're glad you saved some water so you can paint today." Colin beamed as he painted a brightly colored and cheerful picture. When the play session was over, Colin proudly showed his picture to his mother, who promised to hang it up on the refrigerator.

The following week, Colin's mother reported that the school had called to say that Colin's out-of-control behavior stopped the day after his second play session. In subsequent play sessions, Colin's angry play diminished significantly. He no longer trashed the room, and he began to engage for a number of sessions in mastery play. Later, he enacted some family scenes in which the parents were fighting and the kids hid under their beds. This type of symbolic play is often what a child needs to cope in a dysfunctional family.

Variations of CCPT

While CCPT has come a long way since its inception by Virginia Axline, there may be variations from one nondirective play therapist to the next. The important thing is that therapists remain true to the eight guiding principles that Axline originally outlined in her book and to some of the methods she employed. As the CCPT approach has evolved, however, some things have changed since Axline's initial work. Therapists using CCPT today do not take notes during play sessions, and they respond to questions in a more reflective way rather than simply providing information. Therapists also typically do not spend as much time or effort introducing the play materials to child, but allow children to explore the toys in their own way. Most CCPT therapists now sit at a child's level, often on the floor near the child or on child-sized chairs.

Although present-day therapists using CCPT all adhere to Axline's eight principles, there are variations among them in some of the methods they use. As L. F. Guerney (personal communication, 2009) has noted, Virginia Axline did not describe methodologies in great detail in her writings. Subsequent practitioners have had to "translate" her work into the methodologies that have since emerged for CCPT. They have thoughtfully applied principles and methods from Rogerian psychology and Axline's principles, and pieced together information from several other sources. Because of this process, there now exist several different approaches to CCPT—united by Axline's principles, but each with its own unique qualities (see, e.g., L. F. Guerney, 1983, and VanFleet, 2006a, for the Guerney approach; for other variations, see Landreth, 2002; Wilson & Ryan, 2005).

Similarities among these approaches to nondirective play therapy far outweigh the differences, but there are differences. This volume represents the approach developed by the Guerneys as we have described it in the Preface and learned it under the Guerneys' tutelage. It is the culmination of many years of therapy with numerous children in a variety of settings. With stylistic differences in mind, we have shared our rationale for the specific methods described herein, most specifically in Chapter 5 (on CCPT skills) and in Part IV (on practical applications and issues).

PART II

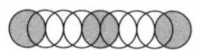

LOGISTICS AND TECHNIQUES

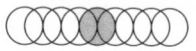

CHAPTER 4

Playroom Set-Up and Logistics

After deciding to conduct CCPT sessions, play therapists have many things to consider in creating an appropriate therapeutic atmosphere for children. These considerations include (but are not limited to) the space to be used, the types of toys to be included, furniture that is appropriate for children, and the logistics of practicing CCPT in their particular setting. It is important to note that CCPT and its family therapy derivative, FT, have been used in a wide variety of settings—including clinics and mental health centers (Ginsberg, 1976; L. Guerney & B. G. Guerney, 1987; L. F. Guerney, 2001; VanFleet, 2005, 2006a), offices of private practitioners (Ginsberg, 1997, 2003; Mandelbaum & Carter, 2003), schools (B. G. Guerney & Flumen, 1970; White, Draper, & Flynt, 2003; Reynolds, 2003), prisons (Adalist-Estrin, 1986; Harris, 2003; Landreth & Lobaugh, 1998; Lobaugh, 2003), residential programs (Ginsberg et al., 1984), early childhood and at-risk programs (Caplin & Pernet, in press; B. G. Guerney, 1969; L. F. Guerney, 1991; Wright & Walker, 2003), domestic violence shelters (Barabash, 2004; Ramos, 2003), and private homes after a parent has learned CCPT skills from a trained FT therapist (B. G. Guerney, 1964; VanFleet, 2005, 2006b; Ginsberg, 1997). Even if a setting does not have a dedicated playroom, it does not take much effort to set up an area that affords a child both sufficient privacy and sufficient freedom to play. It need not be the perfect setting, but CCPT does require that appropriate toys be available for the child and that the need for limits be minimized. This chapter looks at some possibilities and examines what can make some not-so-perfect areas appropriate for CCPT.

Generally, practitioners of CCPT in public clinics or private offices have an office space that they can call their own. Having a dedicated playroom is of course the ideal situation, as the toys and furniture remain in the playroom and the room is always ready for use. In settings such as schools or day care settings, a variety of playrooms or play spaces have been or can be established. These include places such as the school library, an administrator's office, or a corner of a classroom where free-standing bookshelves are used to establish some separateness and privacy from other children in the larger part of the room. One school counselor (C. Mader, personal communication, 1998) began with a makeshift playroom in the janitor's closet when the janitor was not using it, until her successes led to the school district's purchasing a dedicated "play therapy van" she could drive to three different elementary schools!

Obviously, the use of a space that is not dedicated as a playroom requires setting some additional limits, such as keeping children away from parts of the room, items, or furniture not considered part of the playroom. Thus things like papers on a desk, books on a bookshelf, or decorations on a wall will be off limits during the play therapy session. In these settings, the toys often need to be stored away after the play therapy sessions are completed. In a residential facility for developmentally disabled adults, CCPT was successfully taught to the staff of a community living arrangement program. The staff–client play sessions were held in a play area of the living room, and supervisors unobtrusively observed these through open bookshelves that separated the living room and the dining room. In prisons, parents who are incarcerated have been trained in CCPT in a large communal room with a large number of toys placed around it. As each child plays with a parent, an FT therapist supervises the parent in the appropriate CCPT skills. In other cases, prison inmates have learned the principles of CCPT and practiced the skills with each other, taking turns playing the role of the child. Then each inmate has conducted nondirective play sessions with his or her own child each week in a relatively private room when the child comes to visit.

When parents conduct CCPT in their own homes as part of the FT process, the therapist devotes one session in the office to planning an appropriate area in the home for play sessions. Some considerations in the home include setting additional boundaries that may be necessary to protect the home from damage; helping parents understand why televisions, computer games, or other types of technology are not appropriate for their parent–child play sessions; and determining how to handle the use of water as a play medium in the home setting. Most often, parents conducting CCPT sessions at home use a corner of the basement, the family room, or the kitchen as the "playroom" area. In the kitchen, obvious limits need to be set on the use of water, and appliances and cabinets also need to be placed off limits during the play session. In a large area such as a basement, parents are encouraged to use a corner so that there are at least two walls to establish the perimeter of the play session area, and to use either a large area rug, appropriately placed furniture, or masking tape on the floor to demarcate the other limits of the play space. A last resort is a child's bedroom, because this space "belongs" to the child, and the child may resent the disruption of his or her haven. However, one of us (Andrea E. Sywulak) was asked by a single mother (with the children's consent) to observe her home play sessions, which were held in a 6-foot-by-4-foot area of playable space in the children's tiny bedroom. Neither the mother nor the children could determine any other space, as their one-bedroom apartment was very small and extremely crowded with their few pieces of furniture, and the mother slept in the tiny living room area. Ultimately, this very small space with good limit structure was conducive to highly successful outcomes with these two children. Although flexibility and creativity are sometimes needed, obstacles about space can usually be overcome. All of the options described here have been used successfully for CCPT and FT. The most important thing is simply to have a defined space that clearly contains the play sessions.

Playroom Set-Up

The ideal size of a playroom for CCPT is generally 12 feet by 12 feet. As noted above, however, a space as small as 6 feet by 4 feet in a parent's apartment was used successfully. Though it may be hard to believe, very large areas are probably the least conducive to good CCPT. One has to remember that structure and limits play a large role in establishing the appropriate atmosphere for CCPT. In very large spaces, children often feel lost in an area that seems boundless. When children have that sense of boundlessness, they often feel out of control and unable to pull themselves together. This can be most evident on a school playground, where, unless they are given some physical limitations or structure, a number of children with self-control issues will wildly run about and sometimes crash into other students in their frenzy. Although most children with a fair amount of self-control will define their own spatial limits regarding free play in a school yard, a child without good internal controls is relying on the outside world (i.e., adults) to provide the safety that comes with good structure, physical boundaries, and limit setting. The frenzy of such a child can be regarded as a plea for someone to impose limitations that will help the child gain a modicum of self-control. In CCPT, the ideal room size gives the child the freedom to move about and play actively or aggressively, knowing that the play is confined by the structure provided by the walls of the playroom. In order for a child to do effective "work" in CCPT, a sense of safety in the room is paramount. This sense of safety is created by imposing (1) physical structures like walls or clear markings that delineate where the playroom ends, and (2) limits on the child's behavior to let the child know that the therapist will stop him or her if those boundaries are violated.

CCPT therapists can add their own touch to the look of the playroom. For example, some therapists decorate the walls of the playroom with paints in primary colors. Others choose to adorn the walls with murals that will interest the population of children with whom they work. Still others choose to keep the walls neutral, so as to convey a sense that the playroom is a blank slate in which children are free to create their own scenarios. As long as the walls are representative of freedom for all children to express themselves fully and to be who they are, there is no right or wrong décor.

Child-sized furniture is a welcome addition to the CCPT room. It conveys the message that this room is designed for children with their needs in mind. A child can stand at a table that is the appropriate height for painting, drawing, or building a clay model. Or, the child can sit in a child-sized chair, which means that his or her feet are not dangling as they do on most adult furniture. Bookshelves that are no more than four shelves high allow toys to be organized and easily reached. A play sink and stove combination provides a "kitchen" for the child to create food or drink concoctions or pour water from a quart-size pitcher.

A sturdy wooden dollhouse with furniture and miniature dolls gives the child permission to engage in dramatic family play. A blackboard or whiteboard attached to the wall or a free-standing easel will afford the child the opportunity to be the "teacher," leave messages about his or her experiences, create artwork, or draw a target at which to shoot the dart guns. All this furniture is chosen with children in mind and with the intent of letting children know that they are valued in this place.

The CCPT therapist shows acceptance of the child in a physical way by being at the child's level. This means that the play therapist does not hover over the child, but rather sits on the floor or on a child-sized chair to convey acceptance of the child at his or her level. Being at the child's level also makes the therapist more accessible to a child who wishes to include the therapist in play. If a child wants the play therapist to stand up and play Nerf basketball with him or her, for example, the CCPT therapist acknowledges the desire for the therapist to join in the play, and then engages in the play from whatever position the child dictates. Occasionally, an adult-size chair may be introduced into the playroom if the therapist needs it because of pregnancy, recent surgery, or other physical conditions.

The playroom for FT is set up in much the same way, but some adaptations are necessary, especially if FT is done with a group of parents. An observation area, one-way mirrors or observation booths, and other adaptations are discussed elsewhere (VanFleet, 2005, 2006b).

Principles of Toy Selection

In CCPT, much thought is given to the selection and inclusion of toys in the "special room." It is important to remember that toys are chosen on the basis of their variety of uses and significance in eliciting feelings as the children play. Overly structured toys, such as the game of Monopoly, are not considered to be good CCPT toys because there is basically only one thing to do with those toys (e.g., play Monopoly). Similarly, computer or hand-held electronic games are not appropriate for CCPT because children tend to "lose" themselves in these games, barely hearing the play therapist's commentary. Although these types of games may have usefulness in more directive play therapy approaches, they have little to offer in building the relationship between the child and therapist in a CCPT context. Less structured games (e.g., checkers or cards) can be included, as it is easier to use them in multiple and imaginative ways.

Generally, the best CCPT toys fall into five categories: family/nurturance, communication, aggression, mastery, and creative expression. These categories are not mutually exclusive, and some toys fit into more than one category. It does not seem coincidental that three of the toys most frequently chosen by children in CCPT (i.e., the bop bag, dart guns, and water) can fit into at least four of these categories, depending on how a child chooses to use them. VanFleet (2005) has outlined three primary factors to consider in selecting a playroom toy: The toy (1) should be safe for children, (2) should encourage the expression of feelings and play themes, and (3) should allow for imaginative play or projection. Items according to category are listed below, to help a new CCPT therapist accumulate appropriate playroom toys.

Family/Nurturance Toys

Some toys readily permit the expression of family themes or nurturance and attachment-related play.

- Doll family (mother, father, sister, brother, baby)
- Puppet family and/or animal puppets
- Boy and girl baby dolls
- Two life-sized plastic baby bottles
- Doll blanket and crib or basket
- Small paper diapers and wipes
- Dollhouse with furniture
- Kitchen set, including sink and stove
- Child-sized table and chairs

Communication Toys

Some toys are symbolic of human communication and include devices that people typically use to communicate or connect with each other. They are closely related to social relationships as well.

- Telephones, including cell/mobile phones
- Megaphone
- Binoculars
- Two walkie-talkies, preferably ones that actually work

Aggression Toys

By their presence, some toys communicate to children that aggressive play is acceptable, and they permit the expression of aggressive feelings and impulses.

- A 36- to 48-inch inflated bop bag (bags with sand bases last longer than those filled with water)
- Two dart guns with a number of darts
- Two bendable rubber knives
- Small plastic soldiers
- Small plastic dinosaurs
- A 6- to 10-foot piece of rope or jump rope
- An aggressive-looking puppet, such as a wolf, dragon, or "biting" figure
- Foam aggression bats or swimming "noodles"

Mastery Toys

Some toys permit children to achieve developmental mastery, as well as mastery of various dilemmas or problems.

- Plastic quart-size container with 1–2 cups of water
- Water toys, including:
    - Measuring cups
    - Play dishes, pots and pans, and bowls
    - Measuring spoons and play cooking utensils
    - Plastic food items
- Bean bag toss game
- Target for dart guns (easily constructed out of a Lucite sheet)
- Ring-toss game
- Jump rope
- Hula hoop
- Nerf basketball, paddle ball, or baseball
- Bowling pins
- Large checkers
- Deck of cards
- Building toys such as Legos, bristle blocks, or wooden blocks
- Heavy cardboard "bricks"

- Paper towels
- Toss Across

Creative Expression Toys

Some toys permit the expression of a wide range of feelings, hopes, and concerns.

- Dress-up clothes, hats, scarves, fabric pieces
- Masks
- Play money
- Watercolor paints, markers, crayons
- Drawing paper, easel
- Blackboard or whiteboard, chalk or markers, eraser
- Small sandtray/container with miniature toys
- Play-Doh, clay, or other modeling material
- Mirror
- Magic wand
- Cars, trucks, school bus, wooden train set
- Emergency vehicles (fire trucks, police cars, ambulances)
- Medical kit
- Small plastic animals

Toys for Older Children

As children grow and develop, their interest in play materials tends to change. This does not mean that they won't be interested in many of the items on the lists above, as they will often go back and play with these toys. Initially, however, an older child may complain that the toys "are for babies." When this occurs, it is recommended that the child and play therapist have a discussion *outside the play session* about the types of toys that the child would like to see added to the playroom. Sometimes children just want the opportunity to voice their opinion; once their opinions are heard, they may indicate that they are comfortable with the toys already in the playroom, or they may suggest one item they would like to see added. Some children may say that they just want to talk and not play, because they have been to previous therapists who did just that. In such a case, the CCPT therapist reminds the child that "You can *say* or do almost anything you want to in the special room," and that this includes "just talking" if that is what the child chooses to do. Of course, most children who want to "just talk" generally end up playing with the toys, once they get a clearer sense of the freedom of the playroom. When older children do suggest games, it is important to let them know that only games that are not too structured will be considered. Some examples of more appropriate, less structured games include Connect Four, Trouble, Battleship, Candyland, and Sorry. For the sake of keeping cleanup time reasonable, it is generally a good idea to include these games in the playroom only when an older child who requests them is coming. Younger children have a tendency to open games and toss the pieces about rather than playing with them.

Messy Materials

Although it is interesting and valuable to have a wide array of creative toys, such as watercolors, paints, sand, Play-Doh, and water, they can introduce problems for the play therapist. Water is not an issue if the playroom flooring is either linoleum, ceramic tile, or carpet glued down to cement with no padding underneath. Linoleum and tiled floors can be mopped dry, and carpet over cement dries overnight. Some play therapists have a "water corner," which has the play sink and water sitting on top of a flannel-backed plastic tablecloth; in this case, the rule is that "All the water must stay in the water corner or on this cloth." Play-Doh is notorious for sticking to carpet fibers unless it is promptly cleaned up. Clay tends to dry out unless it is carefully returned to an airtight container as soon as the play session is over. All watercolors and other paints should be the washable variety, so that children's clothing does not get ruined, and their use may require some additional limit setting. A rule might be "You can only paint on paper," or if an apron is supplied, "You can only paint while wearing the apron." Sand can also be a cleaning problem unless a rule is stated: "The sand must stay in the tray."

Play therapists must realistically assess their own limits with regard to how much cleanup they are comfortable with. For example, therapists who are "neat freaks" and would be appalled if paint was splattered on the table or floor should probably not include paints in their playroom. Others might decide not to include Play-Doh if their playrooms have high-quality carpeting. It is wiser for play therapists to eliminate a messy toy that gives them distress than to try to fake acceptance and permissiveness. A child almost always can sense a therapist's distress, and subsequently either tests the therapist's limits with that item or avoids playing with the item, perhaps harboring some resentment toward the therapist for providing a toy that feels "off limits" to the child.

Controversy about Aggression Toys

Play therapists often disagree about the use of aggression toys in play therapy. (The broader issue of handling children's aggression during play sessions is covered in a later chapter.) We ourselves continue to use such toys, because we believe that learning to manage aggression is an important and natural part of children's development. Aggression toys help children learn to express and master angry feelings. Most therapists have encountered parents who are opposed to aggression toys, yet admit that even though they don't buy toy weapons for their children, the children use "finger guns" or construct toy weapons out of sticks or various play materials. Including aggression toys in the playroom communicates to children the therapist's willingness to accept aggressive play, albeit within boundaries. Well-reasoned scientific resources are available that examine the myths and clarify this issue, showing that gun play and play fighting actually have social and psychological benefits (Jones, 2002; Mechling, 2008; Pellegrini, 2008).

Louise Guerney once told us a story about a mother in an FT group who could not bear to have guns in the playroom, as her late husband had killed himself with a gun. Dr. Guerney acknowledged and accepted this mother's great fear, and decided it was best to remove the guns during her play sessions. After watching the other parents' play sessions in the group, however, the mother came to realize that with the limit-setting skill, the other children were learning the appropriate use of gun play. She told Dr. Guerney that perhaps if her husband had received the kind of help she was getting for her children, he would have realized that there were more appropriate ways to express himself and to work through his problems. She then asked Dr. Guerney to put the guns back in the playroom during her children's play sessions.

An experienced play therapist (C. Conley, personal communication, 2010) shares a story of a 3½-year-old boy whose mother had been very ill. For three sessions, he and the therapist had to shoot at monsters with the toy guns. The monsters were everywhere. Near the end of the third session of this play, he put down the gun, rubbed his hands together to signify that he was finished, and said, "All done." Subsequently much of his fear and anxiety disappeared, and it seemed as though shooting monsters (which perhaps represented the mother's illness) had helped him gain a sense of control over an uncontrollable situation. Conley reports that this example has been helpful for explaining the symbolic nature of gun use in play sessions to parents.

Arrangement of Toys

To make a playroom inviting to children, there are some important considerations. First, children feel a sense of safety and comfort when there is consistency. This means that the playroom should look very similar each time children come. The toys need to have their own places in the room, even if they are scattered about the room on the floor, set on a table top or bookshelf, or placed in a corner. The blackboard or whiteboard should be erased and the room reset between appointments, so that no evidence of another child's work is left in the playroom.

Second, many children who attend therapy live with a fair amount of chaos in their families. A cluttered or very messy playroom can add to such children's anxiety, as the disorganization resembles the chaos in their lives. Some organization of the toys in a similar manner each time helps children know that the "special room" is separate and distinct from their outside world. It helps to have plastic containers or baskets to hold things like blocks, soldiers, toy trains, or other building toys.

Third, the playroom need not and should not be perfectly tidy. Excessively neat playrooms, with all toys placed in labeled bins or drawers, can give children the impression that free-wheeling play is not accepted—the opposite of the open, inviting atmosphere that the CCPT therapist wants to convey. Instead, playrooms should have some toys in the open and on the floor so that they are immediately accessible. A playroom that is neither messy nor tidy, but somewhere in between, indicates a fun and accepting environment. There should be some open space to permit free movement as well.

Finally, a wide array of toys makes the playroom more inviting. It is important to include at least several toys from each of the five categories mentioned above. Every child will express feelings, work through problems, and build self-esteem in unique ways, so a wide variety of toys enables children to play in the ways that make the most sense to them. In CCPT, therapists never presume to select certain toys in order to elicit the feelings or behaviors on which they think a child needs to work. Toys and play are viewed as the primary vehicles of expression for children. CCPT therapists know that children will find their own way if they are provided with the vehicles they need to get there.

Logistics

The length of CCPT sessions ranges from 30 to 45 minutes. With very young children (i.e., age 3 and under), 20-minute sessions may be appropriate for their developmental needs and attention spans. Generally CCPT sessions are scheduled on a weekly basis. For children with acute problems—such as depression due to the death of a parent, uncontrollable rages, severe sexual abuse, or other intense emotional difficulties—twice-weekly sessions, at least initially, can have a stabilizing effect on the child and give the children more immediate relief from these extreme feeling states. Near the end of therapy, alternate-week sessions may be appropriate in a phased-out discharge process.

CCPT can range from 10 sessions to several years in duration. A review of play therapy practices suggests that the average number of CCPT sessions is 22 (Bratton, Ray, Rhine, & Jones, 2005). Even with mild problems, children typically need at least 10 sessions to become familiar with the therapist and the CCPT process, and then to work through and master their feelings or concerns. In some situations where there is a specific developmental crisis (e.g., the birth of a sibling, the death of a grandparent, or the loss of a pet), CCPT has resulted in successful outcomes in as few as six sessions. For children with severe problems or complex trauma, such as neglect, abuse, or serious attachment problems, CCPT may take from 9 months to several years. These time frames are meant only as approximate guidelines, since the unique needs of children and families necessitate considerable variation in the length of treatment. Specific information about FT logistics is included in the detailed resources about that method (VanFleet, 2005, 2006b).

In many cases, children let the CCPT therapist know when they are ready to terminate treatment. They may begin to ask the play therapist how many more times they need to come, or there may be a decline in their enthusiasm about going into the playroom. Of course, one of the clearest signals that termination may be appropriate is a report from parents or school personnel that significant behavior change has occurred and a child is exhibiting consistently improved behavior and emotional steadiness. Sometimes behavior checklists are completed by parents and teachers at the beginning of treatment and again near the end of treatment, to ensure that therapeutic goals have been met. When it is determined that termination is appropriate, play therapists need to inform children of the discharge plan, with notification that there will be two more play therapy sessions. This advance notification helps children complete the therapeutic process and allows them to bring their relationship with the play therapist to a close. It is also wise to advise parents or other caregivers that critical events sometimes cause children to want to return for a few more sessions, and that it is important for the adults to honor these requests. This shows ultimate respect for children, as it conveys a trust in their ability to know what is needed to maintain the gains made during the CCPT process.

An example of this follows. A play therapist received a call from parents who had participated in FT 2 years prior, asking whether they could resume play sessions with their son following a traumatic event. The mother explained that the week before, an elderly next-door neighbor whom they saw every day did not answer his door. Being concerned, the parents tried to enter the house, but could open only one window to an insufficient height for an adult to crawl through. When their 10-year-old son suggested that he could get through the window, the parents did not stop to think about the possible ramifications and allowed him to do so. Upon entering the elderly gentleman's home, the boy found the man dead on his living room floor. He immediately let his parents in through the front door, and the parents called the police. Although the young boy seemed fine after his grim discovery, he soon began having nightmares about the event and asked his parents if he could resume FT play sessions with them. When the mother called, the therapist asked whether the parents felt comfortable resuming the play sessions independently or whether they preferred to have a couple of refresher sessions in CCPT. They decided to proceed on their own and planned to update the therapist in 2 weeks. Two weeks later, the mother reported that the nightmares had resolved, and she agreed with the FT therapist that approximately 10 parent–child play sessions should be sufficient to help her son completely process this distressing event.

Explaining CCPT to Children

When parents call to initiate CCPT for their children, a common question is "What do I tell my child?" Many children referred for treatment have been punished repeatedly, told they are bad, and/or ostracized by peers, and are languishing in negative self-esteem. Parents sometimes are tempted to tell children that they are taking them to a professional because they have been bad and need to be "straightened out"; in other words, therapy can be presented as a punishment itself. Play therapists, of course, want to start their relationships with children in quite the opposite way. Therefore, the best message that parents or guardians can convey to children is that therapists are people who like children and respect their feelings. When therapists are quite sure that they will recommend FT, they can ask parents to present the situation as follows: "We're going to a special place with a playroom. It's where families go to enjoy each other and learn how to get along better with each other." These presentation options remove the children as the source of the problem and "normalize" the experience to come.

Upon being introduced to the "special room," children may be baffled when they hear, "You can do or say almost anything you want to in here," as this statement alone may stand in stark contrast to the harsh realities of a punitive world. From the very start of treatment, play therapists want children to know that what they do and what they say in CCPT is of utmost importance, and that they can safely explore their feelings and learn to solve their own problems in an atmosphere of acceptance and understanding.

CHAPTER 5

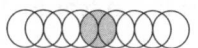

The Four Skills
of Child-Centered Play Therapy

The four basic skills that a CCPT therapist uses are structuring, empathic listening, child-centered imaginary play, and limit setting. The second and third of these skills show children that the therapist understands and accepts their feelings, behaviors, and desires; the first and fourth skills provide the means for setting the tone, ensuring safety, and avoiding or eliminating behavioral problems or conflicts. At any time during a play session, the therapist is using one of these four skills. The skills, when applied properly, provide the atmosphere of safety and acceptance so critical to the child–therapist relationship and to the CCPT process. Each skill is described in detail below, including the rationale for its use, specific methods used by the therapist, and examples. Additional information and suggestions are included to enhance the reader's understanding and use of the skills.

Structuring

The skill of structuring clearly sets the tone and the overall framework for the play session. It helps children understand that CCPT play sessions are different from other playtimes or other interactions in their lives, and it establishes the open and accepting climate needed for therapeutic work. It also helps children realize that they have many choices during the special play sessions, but that the therapist ultimately is in charge, thereby ensuring safety and security. The desired tone is one of invitation into a special place and time wherein children can feel free to be themselves and to explore their ideas and feelings through play.

At its core, the structuring skill opens and closes the play session. The therapist makes statements upon entering the playroom and near the end. These statements are made the same way each time, so children can learn quickly what to expect. In fact, therapists commonly memorize the statements and use them each time in a predictable fashion.

Playroom Entry

Ideally, the therapist makes the room entry statement outside the playroom. If a child enters the playroom first, it is unlikely that the child will hear what the therapist says. If the playroom has a door, the therapist and child stand outside it, with the therapist's hand on the doorknob. In a pleasant voice, the therapist says, "Mike [child's name], this is a very special playroom [or playtime]. You can do almost anything you want in here. If there's something you may not do, I'll let you know." The therapist then opens the door and the session begins.

The therapist does *not* provide the child with a list of the rules at the start. This would set an undesirable negative tone, with a tendency to diminish the child's engagement rather than encouraging it. In essence, stating a list of rules at the start gives this unintended message to the child: "I don't trust you, so I'm going to let you know what the rules are. I'm mostly concerned about keeping control in here." This is not at all a therapeutic message, nor does it create the atmosphere of acceptance essential to CCPT. On a practical level, children rarely break limits during play sessions, making such cautious rule giving unnecessary. For those who do test the boundaries, the limit-setting skill adequately handles such situations.

Children can be so eager to start the play sessions that they sometimes resist the room entry statement, often by impatiently saying, "I know, I know!" Once the therapist believes that a child knows the statement, then the therapist can lightheartedly suggest that the child say it with the therapist or instead of the therapist. After several sessions of this, the therapist can shorten the room entry statement to "Mike, we're going into the special playroom now." It is important, however, to mark the start of the play session, as doing so helps reinforce that this time is different from all other times in the child's life.

Use of Bathroom

It is a good idea for the therapist to suggest that children use the bathroom before each play session. This helps avoid interruptions. A child is permitted one trip to the bathroom during a 30-minute play session, and this time may not be used for other purposes, such as acquiring more water for the playroom, visiting family members in the waiting area, and so on. When the child requests a bathroom break, the therapist says, "You want to go to the bathroom. You may leave the play session just once to use the bathroom." When the child returns, the therapist notes the resumption of the play session by saying, "You're back in the special playroom now."

If a child asks to go to the bathroom a second time, the therapist says, "You have already gone once today. If you leave the room now, our time in the playroom will be over for today." The tone of voice should be firm, calm, and pleasant. The purpose is simply to inform the child of the boundary. If the child then decides to leave, the therapist enforces this rule by closing the playroom door and ending the play session.

Of course, if there are extenuating circumstances (e.g., a child has urinary tract problems), the therapist can be more flexible. Some judgment is required, and if there is a clear physical need, then the therapist can establish a somewhat different boundary for this. On the other hand, if children use the bathroom requests as a means of moving in and out of the playroom at will, they need the therapist to establish the single-bathroom-visit rule firmly. The play sessions must be contained within the playroom in order for therapeutic work to be accomplished. Fortunately, this is a rare occurrence, as most children enjoy the play sessions and show little desire to leave.

Playroom Departure

Like adults, children sometimes need a few minutes to finish something they are working on or to prepare for the transition out of the play session. To accommodate these needs, a therapist gives a child two time warnings prior to ending the session. Typically, the therapist gives a 5-minute and a 1-minute warning that the session is nearing the end.

Five minutes before the end of the session, the therapist says, "Mike [child's name], we have 5 more minutes in the playroom today." One minute before the end of the session, the therapist says, "Mike, we have 1 more minute to play today." At the end of the session, the therapist pleasantly but firmly says, "Mike, our time is up for today. We need to leave the playroom now."

It is quite common in their early play sessions for children to question or resist the idea of leaving the playroom when the therapist gives one of the time warnings. Comments such as "Why?" or "I'm staying," or "I need to finish this!" are ways that children express their unhappiness about ending. In such a case, the therapist reflects the child's feelings—for example, "You're having a good time and hate to see it end." For resistance at the 5-minute and 1-minute warning times, a simple reflection of the child's feelings is sufficient. The time warning does not need to be restated. At the end of the session, however, if the child resists, the therapist reflects the feelings and remains firm about leaving the room, saying pleasantly but firmly, "You hate to go and wish you could stay longer, but we need to leave now." At this point, the therapist's demeanor changes from one of acceptance to one of firmness.

At the end of the session, the therapist also signals the room departure by standing up. Walking out the door and expecting the child to follow is not effective; it is better to stand, give the child a few moments to comply, then walk to the child and say firmly, "I know you want to stay, but it's time to go. Let's go." If the child continues to resist leaving at this point, the therapist can gently take the child by a hand or shoulder and usher him or her out of the room. (We strongly advise therapists to discuss with parents all possible uses of touch, including this one, prior to starting CCPT. Therapists also should have training in the ethics and appropriate methods of touch in child therapy. See Chapter 11 for a fuller discussion.) Once outside the playroom, the therapist can reassure the child that there will be other sessions: "It's hard to leave when you're having fun. I'll see you next time!"

The end of the session is not negotiable. The therapist must be firm and consistent, avoiding any punitive phrases or voice intonations. The purpose is to reassert authority in a kind yet firm manner. This helps contain the play session, assists with the transition, and builds the child's sense of predictability and security. Many children leave the playroom when asked to do so; when resistance does occur it typically happens in the early play sessions, and usually just once or twice before the child understands the process and complies more readily. Therapists should prepare parents for early endings and tantrums, and provide guidance about a coordinated way of handling them should they occur.

Playroom Cleanup

In CCPT, children are not expected to put their toys away. After a child has left, the therapist puts the toys back where they belong. There are several clinical and practical reasons for doing so. First, when children know they do not have to put their toys away, it reinforces for them the special nature of the play sessions. There are few other times in their lives when adults permit them to leave their toys scattered about the room.

Second, children may not play the way they need to if they know they must clean up afterward. For example, children with perfectionistic or obsessive–compulsive characteristics sometimes need to make messes as they become more flexible. Children with serious trauma histories sometimes create jumbles of toys during their play sessions, perhaps reflective of their anger, rage, or confusion. In these situations, children may refrain from engaging in important play if they see a therapist's emphasis placed on cleaning up the playroom rather than on their feelings. Furthermore, the final appearance of the playroom represents these children's therapeutic work for that session. Asking the children to express themselves through their play and then to clean it up afterward is tantamount to asking them to "take back" all that they have expressed and worked through. This invalidates the work that they have done. Along these same lines, cleaning up the toys is a therapist-driven behavior and no longer represents the child-directed nature of CCPT. This violates the most basic principle of nondirective play therapy: The child leads the way. Putting toys away does not show acceptance of the child's expressions. To avoid interference with the child's therapeutic process, it is strongly advised that the therapist tidy the room at the end after the child has left.

Third, a CCPT therapist typically arranges the playroom in a similar manner each time. Asking children to put toys away complicates this process, as they cannot be expected to remember the therapist's blueprint for the toy locations. Telling the children the location for each of the toys would usurp valuable therapeutic time. When children, or even their parents, put toys away, the therapist often must reset the playroom anyway.

Fourth, it is very difficult to enforce a cleanup rule in this type of therapy. What if a child refuses? The therapist has no leverage at this point, and a power struggle only serves to undermine the therapist's authority and all that has been accomplished. It is much easier to enforce the playroom departure, which is an integral part of the therapeutic process.

If, during the final minutes of the play session, the child *chooses* to put toys away, the therapist simply reflects this: "You decided to put some of the toys away." The therapist accepts the child's choice because it is done on the child's own time in the session, but the therapist does not praise or reinforce that behavior. Next time, the child may choose to leave a mess, and the therapist must be accepting of that as well.

Parents often come to therapy worried about their children's forgetfulness or avoidance of such tasks as cleaning up after themselves. The therapist can work with parents to determine whether this is a realistic expectation, an urgent problem to be addressed, or one that can wait while more serious difficulties are addressed. Regardless of the decision, this problem needs to be managed separately from the play sessions. The therapist might consult with parents, for example, to establish a simple behavior plan at home to overcome this difficulty. A therapist should avoid becoming the "disciplinarian" for a child, even though some parents hope that the therapist can "set things straight" with a stern lecture or two. This role is in conflict with the true role of the therapist in CCPT.

Other Structuring Considerations

Several other matters relating to the structuring skill deserve consideration. The use of water and/or sand in the playroom can be very useful therapeutically, but it should be incorporated into the sessions in a way that necessitates a minimum of additional limits. For example, the therapist can control the amount of water that is placed in a container within the playroom. The amount of water can be limited to the amount the therapist can tolerate being dumped onto the floor. If water on the floor is not an option, the therapist can designate a dishpan or tub as the only place for water play. Similarly, if a sandtray is used, it should be filled only to the point where the sand can be easily contained within the tray. If it is too full, then it becomes much more likely that children will be unable to keep the sand in the tray, which is the typical limit placed on sand use.

Sometimes children place toys in their pockets during play sessions. A therapist should not assume that such a child is planning to take the items home, although this may be the case. Instead, the therapist reflects the child's behavior at the moment: "You're putting the car in your pocket." If the child *says* that he or she is going to take it home, the therapist can respond, "You really like that car and wish you could take it home. The toys do need to stay here at the end, but for now, you're putting it in your pocket." Only at the end of the session does the therapist focus specifically on the limit that the toys must stay in the playroom. Infractions are best handled after the child and therapist have left the playroom, perhaps in the therapist's office or waiting area. The therapist can sometimes playfully help the child separate from toys, making it a "game" to empty pockets or reassuring the child that the toys will be in the playroom for use next time. Having a transition routine, where the child gets a small healthy snack or plays in the waiting room play area while the therapist and parent meet, can also help the child readily give up any toys or "transition objects" brought from the playroom. Finally, if the child does not easily yield an item, the therapist can enlist the parent's assistance in returning the toy. If this becomes necessary, the therapist once again reassures the child: "I know that's really important to you, and it'll be here for you to use next time!"

A broader structuring consideration is the cleanliness of toys. Frequently used items that could pass bacteria or viruses to other children, such as toy dishes, should be washed regularly in soap and water. If the therapist permits children to drink water directly from baby bottles in the playroom (sometimes very clinically useful), it is essential to reserve a separate nipple for the use of each child and to wash the bottle itself with soap and water after each session. Attention to cleanliness is important, but it need not become an obsession. If therapists think of other common areas shared by children, such as school or day care spaces, they can determine an appropriate level and frequency of cleanliness for their playrooms. Common sense should be the guide.

Empathic Listening

The skill of empathic listening is the primary means by which therapists communicate their understanding and acceptance to children during CCPT sessions. It shows children that they have their therapists' undivided attention, and that their feelings and needs are heard and accepted. Empathic listening helps therapists see the world from children's point of view while putting their own thoughts and feelings on a back burner during the play sessions. Empathic listening is used whenever a child is playing alone without asking a therapist to play a role. Sometimes, other than structuring, it may be the only skill used throughout a play session if the child chooses to play alone the entire time.

This skill has variously been called "reflective listening," "active listening," or simply "listening skill." In this volume, the preferred term is "empathic listening," because the skill is designed to improve a thera-pist's empathy and attunement to a child. True empathy, whereby one person sincerely tries to see things as completely as possible from anoth-er's point of view, encompasses both an attitude and a skill. A genuine attitude of *wanting* to see the world as the child sees it is essential. The therapist avoids making assumptions about what the child needs, and instead adopts a receptive attitude. Empathic listening requires humil-ity. No matter how much experience one has, or how much one knows about children, truly helping children requires carefully listening to what they have to say—in their words and through their behavior and play. Some of the most competent and experienced CCPT therapists have commented that just when they thought they knew exactly what a child needed, the child showed them otherwise. Listening with the intent of truly understanding is one of the most important tools for any therapist; this is especially true for therapists working with children.

When using empathic listening during play sessions, the therapist puts his or her own thoughts and feelings aside, and pays close attention to the child's verbal and nonverbal behaviors. The therapist notes the child's statements, voice intonation, body language, movements, and any other clues that indicate what the child is experiencing. Then briefly, in his or her own words, the therapist states aloud the main activities in which the child is engaged and any feelings that the child is expressing. For example, if the child is pouring water into some cups, the therapist says, "You're pouring that into the cups." If the child is smiling while pouring, the therapist says, "You're really having fun pouring the water." If the child is frowning while pouring very cautiously, the therapist says, "You're really concentrating on pouring the water. You're trying hard to get it into those cups. You're worried about spilling it." The key is to watch the child's face and reflect the feelings shown there. If a child hits a bop bag with a smile, the therapist might say, "That feels good to you. You like hitting that thing! Pow! Whamo!" If the child has an angry look on his or her face and exclaims, "Take that, you slimebag! That's the last time you mess with me!", the therapist might say, "You're really mad at that guy. You're letting him have it. You're showing him who's the boss! You are WAY more powerful than he is! Pow! Whamo!"

When children play with dolls, puppets, or miniatures and express feelings through the characters, the therapist responds in terms of the characters' feelings. For example, if a child is playing with a toy elephant family and the mother elephant hollers angrily at the baby elephants, the therapist might say, "The mom elephant is really angry and upset with her kids." If the child plays with a bus driving wildly out of control before crashing and rolling, and then indicates that the children inside are crying and yelling for help, the therapist might say in an animated manner as this unfolds, "Yikes! The bus is out of control. No one can stop it! It's going every which way . . . ohh . . . it just crashed, and now the kids inside are yelling for help! They're really scared!"

The technique or method of this skill bears some similarities to the play-by-play commentary sportscasters use to describe a ball game. The therapist makes brief descriptive comments about the play action; this is sometimes called "tracking." When there are emotions present for the child or characters, the therapist also states those feelings aloud.

It should be noted that the therapist's tracking or feeling reflections are made as statements and not as questions. Questions tend to be distracting and can disrupt the flow of the play. Furthermore, the therapist does not "guess" the child's feelings, but instead watches carefully for all verbal and nonverbal signs that convey feelings. The object is to try to understand the child's world and accept the child as he or she is, but therapists should not expect that they will get it right or understand accurately all the time. Human communication is an inexact process. Interestingly, when therapists' empathic listening responses are inaccurate, children typically correct them. This process deepens the therapists' understanding.

For example, 5-year-old Bethann arranged the furniture in the dollhouse, including careful attention to the bathroom. She placed a young female figure on top of the toilet, and then she gave voice to a larger female figure who scolded the younger figure. The therapist, not knowing who or what the figures represented, simply reflected what she saw: "The lady is angry with the girl." Bethann looked at the therapist with a frown and said, "It's not a *lady*. It's the *mom*!" The therapist quickly revised her reflection: "The *mom* is angry with the girl." Satisfied, Bethann continued playing. In this case, the therapist made the most accurate reflection possible, but Bethann did not perceive it as accurate. She then corrected the therapist, thereby clarifying the communication and what she was playing.

A number of other factors are important to ensure the most effective use of empathic listening during play sessions. These are covered below.

Things to Avoid

When therapists use empathic listening, there are a number of common behaviors or statements to avoid. Each of these can be directive or judgmental in nature, and therefore inconsistent with the principles of nondirective play therapy. First, therapists completely *avoid asking questions* during empathic listening. Linguists typically view questions as being directive, in that they carry the expectation that the other person will answer. Also, questions can easily interrupt the flow of children's play. In CCPT, therapists do not ask children any questions about their play or their feelings. With the empathy, attunement, and patience required for empathic listening, therapists can usually determine this information without the need for questions.

CCPT therapists also *avoid giving advice, hints, suggestions, or encouraging statements*. These communications tend to push children toward compliance with whatever adults are suggesting, and are therefore directive in nature. Even simple encouraging statements, such as "I'm sure you can do it!", can negate what a child is requesting or needing at that moment, and therefore can fail to follow the child's lead. These help-giving communications can be appropriate in daily life situations and in other forms of therapy, but their inherently directive nature precludes their use in CCPT.

Related to this, CCPT therapists *do not offer help to children unless asked*. When children struggle with something during a play session, therapists remain in empathic listening mode, saying things like these: "You're trying to put those two pieces together. . . . It's frustrating when they don't go the way you want. . . . You're trying different ways to make it work. . . . You're really proud of yourself for figuring it out!" This approach empowers children to struggle with new tasks, ambiguous situations, and challenges that are created during the play session. When children are free to try to solve their own problems, it becomes part of the growth process and adds to their competence and confidence. If a child asks for help, however, a therapist then gives it. This is following the child's lead. Sometimes children ask for help because they don't know how something works. Sometimes they ask for help because they want to move on to something else and prefer the therapist to take care of something for them. Sometimes they ask for help when they want to feel nurtured or cared for, or to express regressive themes. The key is to follow the child's lead—taking on the helping role when asked, and providing empathic acceptance while avoiding actual helping when the child has chosen to struggle on his or her own.

Carrie, a 9-year-old girl with a 2-year-old brother, provides an example of this. During one CCPT session, her shoe came untied. She sat in a chair and lifted her leg toward the therapist, commanding, "Tie my shoe!" The therapist responded, "You want me to tie it for you," and then did as asked when Carrie nodded. Had this happened in the waiting area or any other environment, the therapist might have said, "I'll bet you know how to tie shoes. Why don't you show me?" Here, in a CCPT session, however, the therapist responded appropriately by following the child's lead. The broader context of this child's life suggested that she enjoyed being treated like a much younger child, perhaps in reaction to the attention her younger brother received. Asking the therapist to tie her shoes might have reflected her own "work" on her sibling rivalry concerns.

Finally, therapists *refrain from giving judgments, such as praise or criticism*, about children's play. Evaluative comments are extremely likely to alter the play. Positive reinforcement is a useful tool in parenting and in other forms of child and adult therapy, but it is a judgment with the power to shift the recipient's behavior, and thus it runs counter to the principles and purposes of CCPT.

Position in the Playroom

Therapists need to convey acceptance and "equivalence" to children in nonverbal ways, at the same time that they are demonstrating acceptance through empathic listening. This means that therapists do not place themselves in a more powerful position than the children. To convey true acceptance and nonjudgment in the relationship, a therapist must enter a child's world, and this means taking a position on the child's level. Standing or placing oneself physically higher than the child emphasizes the adult–child power differential, which can be intimidating to the child. Even subtle messages of dominance must be eliminated, or at least minimized, during CCPT. To do this, a therapist usually sits or kneels on the floor during CCPT. Sitting on a low stool or child's chair can also be appropriate. A therapist who is on the child's level is also more approachable, should the child wish to engage the therapist in the play. While on the floor, the therapist gives the child ample space to play and move around, and backs out of the child's way whenever necessary. On the other hand, the therapist remains physically close enough for the child to show things to the therapist or invite the therapist to engage in imaginary play as desired. Physical positioning needs to demonstrate the same attunement to the child's needs as the therapist's skilled verbal responses do. The therapist moves as needed throughout the session to maintain this positioning vis-à-vis the child.

Handling Children's Questions

Children often ask questions during play sessions. Most common are questions about the toys, the amount of time left in the session, and the rules. Nondirective play therapists initially listen empathically to each question, responding to its intention. For example, if a child asks about a toy, "What's this?", the therapist responds, "You're trying to figure out what that is." If a child asks, "Is this real water?", the therapist responds, "You're surprised to find real water here!" Sometimes the empathic response to the question satisfies the child, and the play continues. Other times, the child persists and verbally or nonverbally continues to question: "Yeah—what is this?" The therapist again empathically listens: "You really want to know. In the special playroom, that can be whatever you want." If this does not satisfy the child, then it is usually obvious that the child requires an answer. At this point, the therapist provides a simple answer, respecting and following the child's lead, and then returns the decision making to the child: "Some people think that's a little desk, but here in the special playroom, you can use it for just about anything you want."

For questions about time left in the session, the same approach is used. When the child asks, "How much time is left?", the therapist responds, "You want to know how much more time." If the child asks again, "But how much time is left?", the therapist responds, "You want to be sure there's enough time. I'll let you know when there are 5 minutes left." If the child persists, "How many more minutes now?", the therapist gives a short answer because the child obviously is asking for one: "There are about 15 minutes left today. It's really important for you to know exactly how much more time you have."

Naming the Toys

There is some debate about whether or not to call a play item by name if a child has not already done so. Reflections can be cumbersome and sound quite unnatural if a therapist avoids naming *any* of the playroom objects: "You're playing with that. Now you've got that other thing. . . . you're putting that thing into the other thing. . . . " Instead, a common-sense approach can be applied. For clearly defined toys or items, it is reasonable for the therapist to call them by name: "You've got the rope, and you're tying a knot in it," "You're pouring the water into the cups." Because of the freedom and acceptance of the play sessions, most children readily correct the therapist if they have something else in mind: "No, it's not water. It's coffee." The therapist then responds to the correction empathically: "Oh . . . you're pouring coffee." On the other hand, for items that are more ambiguous or that can be used in many different ways, the therapist might use more caution in naming them. For example, if the child picks up a strange-looking monster puppet, the therapist might say, "Now you're playing with that one," postponing comments about whether it is a monster or a best friend until the child makes his or her perception of it clearer. The same is true for assigning gender to non-gender-specific toys, such as a bop bag. Unless the child communicates its gender or role, the therapist should stick to neutral reflections, such as "You're really hitting that character!" This is not an area where therapists need to worry excessively. As their relationships with children deepen, the children usually feel much more comfortable about making it clear when the therapists haven't gotten it quite right.

Frequency of Empathic Listening Statements

How often does a therapist comment aloud about a child's feelings and play activities? If the therapist tracks or reflects every one of the child's minute behaviors, it is likely to sound unnatural and perhaps be distracting to the child. If the therapist empathically listens infrequently, the child may notice an unintentional absence of comments for certain behaviors or feelings, and respond to therapist statements as reinforcers rather than as communications of understanding and acceptance. When the therapist speaks sporadically and selectively, the child may perceive the comments as approval and increase certain behaviors—not for the child's own reasons, but in order to gain further approval from the therapist. This is inconsistent with the goals and methods of CCPT.

In one study, VanFleet (1990) found that therapists who responded less frequently in CCPT were much more likely to listen empathically to positive or neutral behaviors and feelings, and to remain silent in response to negative play or feelings, such as aggressive play or angry feelings.

To create the right balance, therapists should use a running but not rote commentary, with reflections of most major changes of play or feelings. Children's responses provide a good guide. If a child continues playing as if a therapist's empathic responses are "background music," the frequency is probably about right. Questions about frequency are often best resolved for new play therapists through professional supervision of their sessions by experienced CCPT practitioners.

Experienced play therapists begin to realize the importance of the timing and frequency of responses by watching and learning from children's reactions. For example, 7-year-old Toby played with the dollhouse, showing how the various family members were preparing for a move (as his family had recently done). The therapist empathically listened: "The mom is moving her things. . . . The boy is moving his things. . . . " As Toby played with the father figure, the therapist hesitated just a bit. Toby stopped playing, looked at the therapist, and said, "But you didn't say what the father is doing!" The therapist hastened to add, "The dad is moving his things now!"

Handling Children's Reactions to Empathic Listening

Most children have little experience with adults' empathically listening to them as is done in the play sessions. They sometimes notice or even resist this different way of talking. Therapists need to be prepared for children who say, "Quit repeating me!" or "Why are you talking like that?" or "Be quiet!" Even highly experienced CCPT therapists get such responses sometimes.

The first consideration is whether or not a therapist's empathic responses sound natural. Is the therapist starting each comment the same way, such as "Sounds like you're happy . . . ," "Sounds like you're upset about that . . . ," and so on. Is the therapist using a flat or incongruent voice intonation? Is the therapist using patronizing phrases, such as "What I hear you saying is . . ."? To correct such problems, the therapist needs to focus on varying his or her empathic responses and on using an interested intonation that is also consistent with the feeling being reflected. Observing their own play sessions on video, preferably as part of supervision, can help therapists develop this skill so that it sounds much more natural.

When a child comments on a therapist's reflections, the first step is to show acceptance through further empathy: "You noticed that I'm talking funny." Sometimes this might be the end of the child's reactions, and play resumes. At other times, the child might continue, "Why do you talk like that?" At this second level, the therapist can offer a brief, benign explanation: "It really sounds weird to you. Well, that's just the way I pay attention in the special playroom." For many other children, this type of response suffices. Still, there are others who continue to react, often by asking the therapist to change: "I don't like it. Quit doing that." Because the child leads the way in CCPT, the therapist reflects and complies: "You want me to stop it. Okay." The therapist then remains quiet, avoiding further tracking statements and reflecting only the feelings present in the play. Typically, the therapist does this for the remainder of the session, and returns to the normal use of empathic listening in the next session unless the child indicates the need for adaptation once again.

Congruence

Most of the time, when therapists genuinely care about children's feelings and points of view, it shows in their nonverbal communications without much conscious thought. Empathic listening is a complex skill, however, and it takes time to develop it into a natural response. Not only must one make brief statements about the play and the expressed emotions; one must also use voice intonations and body language that are congruent with the words being spoken. Words, intonation, and body must all express the same thing in concert. Perhaps the most important way to ensure this is to adopt an attitude that *genuinely* seeks to see the world through the child's eyes. Attitude is vital, because the inside must match the outside; there is no room for duplicity or "faking it."

In addition, it is vital for therapists to maintain an awareness of their own feelings during play sessions. When therapists' feelings of discomfort arise, they have two primary courses of action: to work on their reactions until they are no longer incompatible with being nondirective, or to set a limit on the behaviors that elicit those reactions. CCPT therapists rarely verbalize to children their own feelings or reactions to the play, because of the power differential that exists between adults and children, and the consequent likelihood that children will feel the need to respond to the adults' feelings (thereby leading to adult-centered rather than child-centered interactions). Instead, the therapists strive for congruence and transparency by the manner in which they handle their own reactions and feelings. They neither "grin and bear it" nor pretend that the feelings do not exist. They deal with them directly in a manner that allows them to retain the child-led focus of the play sessions.

For example, Melanie was a new play therapist. She felt quite anxious whenever children engaged in aggressive play, such as hitting the bop bag or pretending to kill off the "bad guys." With the help of her supervisor, she was able to process her underlying fears that she was contributing to the children's behavior problems rather than treating them. She eventually learned to reframe her thinking, seeing the play as more indicative of the children's expressions of distress and their therapeutic work. With this reframing, she became much more comfortable with aggressive play. She also explored with her supervisor where the boundaries lay between acceptable aggressive play and that which could cause damage. This helped her set limits more decisively when needed, added to her own sense of safety in the playroom, and helped her become comfortable with aggressive play. She realized that her responses were not congruent with her need to be accepting, and then she took the necessary steps to achieve congruence.

Intensity and Depth of Empathic Listening Responses

Therapists need to listen empathically to the deepest level of feeling that children express. When a child expresses strong emotions of hate or disgust, for example, it is insufficient for the therapist to respond, "You're upset." With words and intonation, the therapist needs to capture the feeling at its core: "You are *furious!*" or "That makes you really, really *mad!*" A CCPT therapist always looks for the essence of the feeling being expressed, even if a child uses no words to express it. Matching responses to the child's affect adds to the congruence of empathic listening, while conveying to the child that the therapist truly understands and accepts what is being expressed.

For example, Marcie was 4 years old when she was in a car accident that injured her mother and father. During CCPT, she often created car crashes and then rushed the victims to the hospital in the toy ambulance with a great sense of urgency, although she spoke very little. Throughout this scene, the therapist reflected what was happening, but also the feelings beneath the surface of Marcie's play: "There's a bad wreck. They're trying to get them to the hospital really fast. *Really, really* fast. They're worried about the hurt people. They want to get them the help they need!"

A therapist empathically listens to the *intentions* of a child's play as well. The child may not say it directly, but if it is *implied* in the play, the therapist can reflect this. For example, 9-year-old Ben was referred for being oppositional at home and school. He frequently tested the limits in the play sessions, often with a mischievous expression on his face. In one session, he broke five different limits and looked to see the therapist's reaction each time. The therapist set limits appropriately and then reflected, "You're trying to see what the rules are in here. You're wondering how I might react when you break the rules." This response reflected what Ben seemed to be saying with his behavior and facial expressions.

Summary reflections are also permissible. When children play repetitively, or their play clearly reflects a pattern or sequence, the therapist can reflect at this level: "You're pulling out all the red blocks," or "Now you have the boy puppets in one pile and the girl puppets in another pile," or "You're seeing if you can get the ring on the post from farther and farther away." It is best to wait until a sequence is nearly completed before making these types of summary reflections.

Child-Centered Imaginary Play

The skill of child-centered imaginary play is designed for times during the play sessions when a child asks a therapist to play an imaginary scene or role. This offers another way for the therapist to enter the child's world and learn more about the child's perspective, feelings, and experiences. When a child asks the therapist to adopt an imaginary role, the therapist does so, but in a manner that follows the child's lead as completely as possible. The therapist uses the child's verbal instructions as well as nonverbal cues to play roles as the child wishes. In many ways, effective imaginary play that follows the child's lead is another form of empathic attunement: The process offers another avenue to convey understanding and acceptance to the child.

With child-centered imaginary play, the therapist accepts and acts out various roles as assigned and directed by the child. The therapist does not initiate such play until the child invites it. In essence, the child is the director of the imaginary scene, as well as an actor/actress in it.

The therapist is an actor/actress under the child's direction, playing the part as the child determines. The therapist uses various facial expressions, "voices," actions, and sometimes props, puppets, and costumes in playing the part, but always attends to and follows the child's wishes in playing the role. Some children are very specific about what they want, telling the therapist exactly how to move and talk; other children give few instructions, leaving the therapist to surmise what is desired.

The therapist no longer needs to use empathic listening when using the child-centered imaginary play skill, although it is sometimes possible to do so. At no point should any use of empathic listening interfere with the role play, however; if there is doubt, the therapist continues in the imaginary role as long as the child desires. Therapists who become adept at imaginary play convey the same empathy and acceptance as in empathic listening, but do so through the accuracy and attunement of their role playing. Only when the child returns to solitary play does the therapist return solidly to the empathic listening skill.

Playing the Role as the Child Wishes

When playing a role, the therapist watches the child carefully for any signs or clues about what the child wants the therapist to do. Many times, children will correct the therapist's portrayal if it is not what they intended. Playing roles often requires animation and expressiveness, such as using gruff voices, screams, hiding, acting surprised, or running around the room. A child may also dress the therapist in costumes that may look or feel silly. The therapist will do well to play these roles as realistically and playfully as possible, but should stop short of doing anything with the intention of entertaining the child. The purpose, as always, is to follow the child's lead.

For example, 7-year-old Tommy picked up some play money and handed it to the therapist, saying, "You're gonna be the bank lady, and I'm gonna be the robber!" The therapist empathically listened to the role assignment—"I'm the bank person, and you're a robber"—and then assumed the role, laying the money out in front of her as if she were a bank teller. Tommy picked up some toy weapons and put on a mask, approached the therapist, and demanded, "Give me all your money! No funny business! And don't try to call the police!" The therapist gasped, put her hands in the air, and in a wavery voice said, "Okay, Mr. Robber, sir, here's all my money. Please don't shoot!" Then, because of the therapist's sensitivity to Tommy's nonverbals and intentions with the play, she turned aside and pretended to call the police, whispering, "Is this the police? There's a robber here!" Tommy smiled briefly and then roared back, "I told you not to call the police. Now sit there and listen, or I might have to shoot you!" The therapist wore a frightened expression: "Okay, Mr. Robber, sir. I see you really mean business. I'll do whatever you say!" As she sat there timidly, Tommy whispered further instructions to her: "Try to call the police again." She did so, Tommy roared at her again, and their play continued. Tommy's intention was to be the character in control. The therapist read this accurately and played her role in a manner that allowed this to unfold. Her sensitivity to *all* of his communications, both verbal and nonverbal, led her to play the role just as he wished her to.

When children give few instructions about the imaginary play, the therapist enters the role and plays it in a rather neutral manner until more information defines the role better. For example, if a child pretends to be cooking and says, "I'm the mom and you're my little girl," the therapist does not have much information. In this case, the therapist might assume a little girl's voice and say, "Hey, Mom, what're you cooking for us? I'm hungry." Usually more clues about what the child wants follow, such as when the child serves the meals and says, "You have to eat your veggies before you have ice cream. *All* your veggies!" The child's nonverbals are likely to provide further information that might lead the therapist to say in the little girl role, "Yuck! I want ice cream. Do I *have* to eat all the veggies? They're yucky." Again, the child's reactions help determine the further development of the role.

Asking Questions

During child-centered imaginary play, the therapist may ask questions *as the character* if it makes sense for that character to ask questions. However, the questions should be part of the role and should never be intended to gather more information. For example, 12-year-old Jamie asked the therapist, Ed, to pretend to be a teacher and she would be the student in geography class. The teacher was to test her knowledge of state capitals. Ed stood before her and in his most professorial voice said, "Okay, Ms. Jamie, can you tell me the capital of New York . . . That's fine. Now what about Colorado?" In this case, the therapist-as-teacher's questions were within the role and were appropriate.

Other than this use of questions *within* a role, it is best if the therapist avoids asking questions *about* the role, as questions tend to have a leading effect (i.e., to create the expectation of an answer). Children sometimes stop their play entirely when asked questions about it. More importantly, a therapist's questions often interrupt the flow of a child's imagination, because the child must stop one mental process (the non-verbal, imaginative one) in order to answer the therapist's question via a completely different mental process (a verbal, cognitive one). Children often do not plan their play out in detail, and probably not in words; it simply unfolds from one moment to the next. This spontaneity is the essence of play. Having to provide details or explanations to the therapist distracts a child from the process. Furthermore, the context of the play usually gives sufficient clues about the type of role the child wants the therapist to assume. It is less intrusive to take on the role and watch for reactions. It is preferable to stay within the metaphor of the imaginary play and avoid asking for unnecessary explanations that risk leading the play.

On rare occasions, children ask therapists to play roles about which they have absolutely no information or ideas. Perhaps a child tells a therapist, "I'll be King Soonoboono, and you'll be Queen Gabbadabba." These may be characters created by the child or drawn from a story or cartoon with which the therapist is unfamiliar. When the therapist is *totally* lost about the intended role, it is acceptable to ask in a stage whisper, "How does Queen Gabbadabba act?" Such questions should be kept to a minimum, just to obtain enough information to start the role play.

Limit Setting

The limit-setting skill is used to keep both the child and therapist safe during play sessions. It also establishes the therapist's authority when needed, provides a sense of security, protects valuable toys and property, and helps the child become more responsible for his or her actions. Limit setting helps children learn that they are responsible for what happens to them if they choose to break a limit after they've been previously warned and informed of the consequences. This skill provides the necessary boundaries for the play sessions.

The number of limits is kept to a minimum. This preserves an open atmosphere that permits relatively free expression of feelings, so that the sessions have maximum therapeutic value. Minimizing the number of limits also increases children's chances of complying with them.

When limit setting is needed, it takes precedence over all other skills. Therapists permit much room for exploration during play sessions, but they are ultimately in charge. They exert their authority in a calm, firm manner when it is needed.

The limits in CCPT differ from those in daily life because of the therapeutic nature of the play sessions. Open expression of feelings, perceptions, and experiences is critical to the process. By nature, daily life entails many additional security concerns not present in the microcosm of therapy; it is also where children must learn appropriate ways of interacting with their families and friends in different settings, such as school and community. By necessity, there are more rules in daily life. Children, from an early age, are very good at distinguishing different rules in different environments. Therapists might wonder whether there are "spillover effects" from the play sessions—that is, whether children try to take greater liberties at home after the child-directed play sessions. In actuality, this is rare. It seems that when children have an opportunity to express their wishes, impulses, worries, and distress in a special environment, and when they feel understood and accepted for this, they become less likely to push the limits in other environments. Furthermore, when children have been referred because their behaviors are out of control, or they are controlling of others or in inappropriate situations, the play sessions provide a way to redirect their control needs. Instead of trying to control their parents, their friends, or their pets in ways that create problems, they learn through the play sessions how to control something without adverse effects: their play. In the rare cases when children's home behaviors worsen in conjunction with CCPT sessions, the therapist works with parents to pinpoint probable causes and helps them determine a course of action to contain and eliminate the exacerbated behaviors.

Limits are set during CCPT on *imminent* behaviors that are likely to be unsafe or destructive. The therapist sets limits on those behaviors that are unsafe in real time—in actuality. Limits should not be set on the content of the play, the children's imaginary scenarios, or the things children say. All of these represent the children's therapeutic work. Their play choices and themes are their ways of communicating with the therapist, and therefore must be permitted as part of the therapeutic process. Only behaviors that actually result in destruction or are potentially unsafe are curtailed.

Limits set during play sessions vary, depending on the physical facility, but they often include the following:

- Nothing should be thrown at windows, mirrors, or cameras.
- Crayons or markers should not be used on walls, furniture, or blackboards/whiteboards.
- Sharp items and hard-soled shoes should not be poked, thrown, or kicked at the bop bag.
- The child may not leave the room except for one trip to the bathroom.
- There should be no destruction of valuable toys or mass destruction of toys.
- Nothing that is likely to result in injury to the child or therapist should occur.
- Hard toys should not be thrown at the therapist.
- Sand needs to stay inside the sandtray or sandbox.
- With the exception of shoes, the child's clothing should stay on.
- The child may not put toys into his or her mouth, unless they are specifically made for this purpose (such as the child's own personal baby bottle nipple).

Therapists sometimes have personal limits that become part of the CCPT process. For example, if a therapist feels uncomfortable about being blindfolded, he or she may set a limit on that. When children ask the therapist to behave in a manner that is uncomfortable or inappropriate, the therapist simply says that he or she is not able to comply. A 9-year-old girl, Zoe, had a history of sexual abuse. Her play sessions began to reflect trauma themes, suggesting that she was working through some of the issues of her abuse. During one session, she lay down on the floor and asked the therapist to pin her hands down on the floor over her head. The therapist sensed that this play, though related to her trauma work, had a strong likelihood of triggering a flashback or other adverse reaction for Zoe. Because the therapist would never hold a child down forcibly anyway, he said, "You want me to hold your hands down, but I don't ever hold people down. You can play almost any other way, though." After some initial disappointment, Zoe selected a puppet to be placed loosely over her hands so that she could continue her play.

As discussed above in the section on the structuring skill, therapists state the limits only when children actually break them or when an infraction seems imminent. When limits are needed, however, therapists need to state them and enforce them firmly and consistently. Children quickly learn from this that their therapists mean what they say, and limit-testing behaviors usually resolve in a matter of one or two sessions.

Consequence

During play sessions, the same consequence is used for any limit that a child pushes too far (i.e., for any limit that the child goes beyond three times). The consequence is that the child must leave the playroom, and the session ends. Despite whatever inconsistencies children have experienced in other environments, this is a consequence that is meaningful for them and that clearly demonstrates the therapist's authority when needed. Meaningful consequences that are consistently enforced establish the safety and sense of security that many children need, even though they do not like it. In reality, it is rare for children to push a limit as far as the consequence, but it does happen sometimes. It is exceptionally rare for children to return and push limits that far again. This is true of children with severe behavioral difficulties as well. The limit-setting process and the firm, predictable consequence help contain children's behavior while helping them develop more responsibility for their actions and greater self-regulation. If the playroom becomes unsafe for either a child or a therapist, it is no longer therapeutic. Limits and enforcement of the consequence are critical for CCPT sessions to retain the physical and emotional safety that is essential to the process.

Limit-Setting Process

A three-step sequence of stating the limit, giving a warning, and enforcing the consequence is used during CCPT. This allows the child two opportunities to self-correct before the therapist intervenes. This three-step process is completed for each new, different limit that is broken. The three steps are outlined below.

1. *Stating the limit.* When a child breaks or obviously is about to break one of the playroom limits, the therapist states the limit in a brief, clear, specific manner. The tone of voice should be pleasant, but firm and assertive. The therapist uses the child's name to gain his or her attention, and if there is time, reflects the child's desire to perform the prohibited behavior. The therapist then states the limit and restructures

for the child so that he or she can redirect the play. For example, the therapist might say, "Annie [child's name], you'd like to shoot the dart gun at me. Remember I said I'd let you know if there's something you may not do. One of the things you may not do here is point or shoot the dart gun at me when it's loaded. But you can do just about anything else." A shorter version, if one is needed to stop an imminent action, might be this: "Annie, one of the things you may not do is point the gun at me when it's loaded. But you can do just about anything else." If needed, the therapist can also signal the limit by raising a hand in a "stop" position, especially if this is needed for protection from flying objects! After stating the limit and the redirection statement, the therapist returns to empathic listening or imaginary play, depending on what the child is doing.

2. *Giving a warning*. If the child engages in a behavior for which the therapist has already stated the limit earlier in the session (i.e., this is the second time the behavior has occurred in the same session), the therapist gives the child a warning. To do this, the therapist restates the limit and then informs the child what will happen if the child breaks the limit again. This allows the child to choose whether or not to risk the consequences. After the warning is given, the therapist restructures once again so the child can redirect his or her play. For example, the therapist says, "Annie, remember I told you that you could not point or shoot the gun at me when it's loaded. If you point or shoot it at me again, we will have to end the playtime today. You may do just about anything else." As before, the therapist returns to empathic listening or imaginary play, as the child's behavior determines.

3. *Enforcing the consequence*. If the child breaks the same limit for the third time that day, the therapist must enforce the consequence. To do this, the therapist restates the limit and then carries out the consequence as stated in the warning. A pleasant but firm voice is used. The therapist guides the child out of the room if necessary, following the same procedures described for playroom departure in the section on the structuring skill. This procedure helps children learn that they are responsible for their choices and behaviors and for the outcomes associated with them. During this third limit-setting step, the therapist says, "Annie, remember I told you if you pointed the dart gun at me again, we would have to leave the playroom today. Since you chose to point it at me again, we have to leave now. Right now." There is no negotiation at this point.

In subsequent play sessions, the therapist starts with step 1 only if it is the first time the child has broken that particular limit. If the child has broken the limit in a recent play session, the therapist starts at the warning step and proceeds to the enforcement step if necessary. The therapist uses judgment about the child's age and level of understanding when handling limits in this way. For example, for a 3-year-old child, the therapist might decide that it's important to start at step 1 again if the child is likely to have forgotten the previously stated limit.

Redirection after Broken Limits

When therapists state limits and give warnings, they end with a statement to help children redirect their play: "But you can do almost anything else." Sometimes there is a temptation to tell children precisely what they can do instead of the limited behavior, such as "You may not shoot the dart gun at me, but you can shoot it at the wall over there." These specific types of redirection statements should be avoided. Axline's fifth principle (1969, p. 73) is that "The therapist maintains a deep respect for the child's ability to solve his own problems if given an opportunity to do so. The responsibility to make choices and to institute change is the child's." When a therapist sets a limit, the therapist is thwarting the child's desire to do something—in essence, creating a "problem" for the child. This therapeutic problem is *not* about how to use the toys properly; it is about how the child will handle the feelings that caused him or her to violate the rule. If the therapist tells the child precisely what he or she can do instead, it is the *therapist* who is solving the problem and giving advice to the child. Using a more general redirecting statement (such as "You can do almost anything else") is much preferred, because it leaves the problem solving in the child's hands. If the therapist tells Annie where she can shoot the gun, the therapist has removed much of the responsibility for solving the problem (in Annie's case, how to release aggressive impulses safely) from the child.

Self-Regulation in CCPT

The three-step limit-setting process of CCPT is valuable in helping children develop self-regulation, both emotionally and behaviorally. When a child behaves in ways that are not permitted, the therapist stops the child. Very often, limited behaviors are aggressive to a point where they could be dangerous or destructive. The child has the impulse; the therapist stops the mode of expression; and the child must come up with an alternative way to manage or express the impulse. Because children enjoy being in the playroom and the consequence is leaving the playroom if they continue to violate the rules, they become motivated to find alternative ways of handling their impulses, desires, emotions, and behaviors. This relates to the value of general redirection statements, as noted just above. The nonspecific redirection puts the responsibility for change in the children's hands, and eventually they learn more effective and acceptable means of dealing with their feelings and impulses.

Setting Limits for Behaviors, Not Intentions

Sometimes adults excuse children's inappropriate behaviors because the children "didn't really mean it," or they "didn't intend for that to happen." Children quickly learn that they can use this reasoning to avoid consequences: "I didn't mean to hit you. The toy just bounced over that way." Nevertheless, to help children develop responsibility for their choices and behaviors, therapists need to place the boundaries on the potentially bad *behaviors* rather than on what they believe were the children's intentions. Because children are given two chances to correct their behaviors in this limit-setting process, therapists must be clear and consistent in placing limits on any behavior that could result in injury or destruction. Even if a child does not intend to hit a therapist, a hard resin dinosaur toy will hurt just as much when it hits the therapist's face. The example that follows shows how even very young children without good motor control can learn to rein in their behaviors so that they are safe.

TJ was 3½ years old and referred because his behavior was out of control both at home and at the day care facility he attended. Effective limits had been largely absent from his life. TJ also had some developmental problems resulting in poor motor control. During a play session, TJ began throwing the wooden blocks around the playroom. Before long, the blocks reached the therapist, who was sitting about 6 feet away from him in the small playroom. It did not appear that TJ was aiming for the therapist; he was throwing blocks in all directions. The therapist realized that TJ's behavior could result in injury, however, so he set the limit: "TJ, I know you're having fun throwing the blocks, but you may not throw them in my direction. You can do just about anything else, though." TJ continued throwing the blocks around the room. Again some of the blocks bounced toward the therapist, who moved to the second step of limit setting: "TJ, remember I told you that you cannot throw the blocks in my direction. If that happens again, we will have to leave the special playroom. You can do just about anything else, though." TJ stopped for a moment and responded, "I didn't mean to!" The therapist replied, "You want me to know that you didn't do it on purpose, but that's still the rule here. You can do just about anything else that you wish in here." TJ then decided to throw the puppets around, and no further limits were required.

In this example, TJ did not have the coordination to control where the blocks were going. When his behavior became potentially dangerous, the therapist rightly set a limit. Even though TJ was not deliberately trying to hit the therapist, he needed to learn to adjust his behavior so that everyone stayed safe. He was capable of making the decision to alter his play rather than risk the end of the playtime.

Multiple Limits

It is not common, but sometimes children will break several different limits in a play session. Rosie, an 8-year-old child with serious trauma and attachment problems, broke four different limits in her first play session: She tried to break the bop bag with a hard plastic magic wand; she threw a toy at the therapist; she tossed a handful of sand across the room; and she tried to climb onto a shelving unit that would have collapsed under her weight. In these rare limit-testing cases, the therapist starts at the first step of limit setting with each new limit. In Rosie's case, the therapist set four different limits, all at step 1. Had Rosie thrown sand a second time, for example, the therapist would have moved to the warning stage for that broken limit. Interestingly, even though Rosie mightily tested the limits, she never pushed any single limit to the point where the play session ended. This pattern of behavior also permitted the therapist to offer an intention reflection after the fourth limit was set: "You want to see what the rules are like in here and how I'm going to react." Rosie actually smiled when the therapist reflected her feelings in this manner.

Clear Limits

When setting limits, a therapist must use clinical judgment about whether a child fully understands the limit. The language used for setting limits must be developmentally appropriate for the child: The more behaviorally specific the limit is, the more likely it is to be understood. "You may not make a dent in my skin" is a better limit statement than "You may not hurt me" for a child who is aggressively punching a toy needle into the therapist's arm while playing doctor. "You may not touch me below this button on my jacket" (said while pointing at the button) is clearer than "You may not touch my private parts." When a therapist is first learning to use the limit-setting skill as outlined here, it can be useful to memorize the first and last parts of the limit, thereby leaving only the specific behavioral description to be filled in: "_____ [child's name], one of the things you may not do is _____ [specific behavior goes here], but you can do almost anything else."

Are You Really Being Nondirective?

Many questions arise for new CCPT therapists. When there is any doubt about a situation, it is very important to think about Axline's eight principles (see Chapter 3) and see what they suggest. If doubt persists, a consultation with an experienced CCPT supervisor is in order.

Because therapists' attitudes, cognitions and behaviors need to be congruent when they are using CCPT, they need to monitor their motives and other cognitions during play sessions. The following checklist provides a tool to consider whether or not your motives have strayed from the nondirective stance needed in CCPT. If you are tempted to . . .

- Find out a little more information about the child's play . . .
- Alter something to see how the child might react . . .
- Use the moment to try to teach the child something . . .
- Help the child just a little to relieve his or her struggling . . .
- Let the child know how much you like what he or she is doing . . .
- Encourage the child to do something more independently . . .
- Reassure the child when he or she is feeling afraid or sad . . .
- Help the child move forward a bit more quickly . . .
- Calm the child down when he or she is expressing anger or rage . . .
- Tell the child what to do instead of what he or she is doing . . .
- Give a little hint that might help the child succeed . . .

. . . then you may be on the verge of leading the play rather than following the child's lead. Instead, try refocusing on the child's thoughts, feelings, motives, and themes. If this is difficult, supervision may be indicated. Some of the items on this list are used at times in more directive play therapy approaches, but they violate the basic principles underlying CCPT, and it is a good idea for therapists to be cognizant of their own internal processes during any type of work with children.

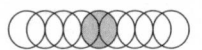

CHAPTER 6

Recognition and Interpretation of Play Themes

After a play session has concluded and the child has departed, the therapist considers possible meanings of the child's play during the session. To do this, the therapist considers the play themes that were expressed. "Play themes" are patterns or instances of a child's play that appear to have meaning for the child. Play themes may be clinical and/or developmental in nature. Therapists must exercise caution when interpreting children's play themes, in order to avoid either underestimating their importance or reading too much into them. There are many times when the meaning or relevance of children's play remains a mystery, and sometimes it represents nothing of psychological importance—it's just play. In CCPT, as long as a therapist is skillfully applying empathy, attunement, and acceptance, it is not critical if the therapist fails to grasp the deeper meanings of the play at any given moment. The safety and acceptance of CCPT play sessions help children work through their concerns and dilemmas even when therapists do not fully understand the meanings of particular segments of the play. Trying to understand play themes is valuable nonetheless, for this understanding yields greater attunement and improved empathy in subsequent play sessions, helps therapists provide general information to parents and caregivers about the play sessions, and alerts therapists to possible child concerns they have not yet recognized.

Recognition of Play Themes

There are several ways to recognize play themes. The following signals alert therapists that play may have particular meaning for children.

• *Repetition.* When children select the same toys or play activities multiple times, it is likely that these choices are meaningful.

• *Similar activity with different toys.* When children engage in the same or a similar activity but use different toys, such as using a variety of items to set traps for ghosts, this activity is likely to represent a play theme.

• *Intensity and focus.* Sometimes children play with great intensity. This is seen in their facial expressions, voice intonations, and body movements. They also may focus much more intently on some aspects of their play. The play may be noisy or quiet, but the essential feature is that a child is very focused on what he or she is doing. What the child pays the most attention to is likely to be most meaningful to him or her.

• *Play sequences that occur in several play sessions.* When children's play choices or sequences are similar across several play sessions, it is probably a sign of a play theme. The play may be very much the same each time or may suggest variations on a theme.

• *Sudden changes.* Sometimes children stop their play sequence suddenly, or they quickly and noticeably shift focus to something quite different. Sudden changes can happen at any time during play sessions, and they are sometimes associated with the 5-minute or 1-minute warnings near the end.

• *Continuing play from the prior session.* Sometimes children refer to their play from the prior session, indicating that they wish to pick up the thread of that play and continue with it. They may even reestablish the playroom as it looked at the end of the prior session and then continue with the play as if it had never been interrupted.

• *Emotional tone.* Sometimes the emotional tone (i.e., the overall sense or feeling) of the play session suggests that the play is meaningful for the child.

Critical Considerations in Understanding Play Themes

Having a strong knowledge of child development, and knowing what characterizes "normal" child play at different stages of development, are very important for identifying and understanding play themes during CCPT. It is valuable for therapists to become familiar with a wide range of children's play, in order to gain perspective and to keep in touch with typical play activities, toys, and themes.

Much of children's play in CCPT reflects developmental tasks and themes. Not all themes relate to mental health or clinical issues. For example, a 5-year-old's continuous pouring of water back and forth between containers is more likely to reflect developmental mastery than obsessive–compulsive disorder. A therapist should always think about the child's physical, social, emotional, cognitive, and moral developmental stages when considering play themes and their meanings for the child. A strong acquaintance with the child development work of Piaget, Erikson, and Kohlberg is essential.

Play therapists look for meanings in the *patterns* of children's play and must avoid drawing any firm conclusions from single occurrences of play. CCPT therapists learn to accept the unknown and have patience. Enthusiasm for interpretation must be tempered with a single-minded focus on the child's process. Frequently patterns emerge over the course of several play sessions, and meanings become clearer as a result. Occasionally a therapist never really knows what a segment of play means to a child, but the child's problems resolve nonetheless.

To ensure an accurate understanding of children's play themes in CCPT, therapists should explore alternative explanations of the play, reserving their conclusions until patterns emerge to confirm one of their "working hypotheses." For CCPT novices, play therapy supervision can greatly assist them in developing the abilities to recognize and interpret play themes.

Thematic Stages in CCPT

L. F. Guerney (2001) has identified relatively predictable stages in children's play in CCPT. These stages have been noted so frequently that therapists should be aware of them. Not all children go through them, nor are they always manifested in the sequential order presented here, but they are quite common. Stage duration varies considerably among children. The stages refer to the predominant nature of a child's play during CCPT sessions, but they are not intended as exclusive descriptions of all that the child is playing and expressing in any given session. The four stages are called "warm-up," "aggressive," "regressive," and "mastery" in valuable articles by Nordling and Guerney (1999) and L. F. Guerney (2001); they are summarized below.

Warm-Up Stage

The warm-up stage occurs at the start of CCPT. During their early play sessions, children adjust to the playroom, the freedoms it represents, and the therapist's comments and behaviors. Although it is common for children to explore the playroom without focus on any particular activity, some children may select one toy or area and stay there, seemingly uncomfortable with exploration. Limit setting can occur as other children adapt to the new environment, while still other children remain on their best behavior. The warm-up stage also includes rapport building (i.e., the development of initial trust in the therapist and the process).

Aggressive Stage

As children become more trusting and comfortable in the CCPT sessions, they usually relax, and their behavior shifts. Nordling and Guerney (1999) note that aggressive behaviors develop and peak during this period for children with either internalizing or externalizing problems. Inhibited children's aggressive play can be relatively quiet, but it represents a change for them. For instance, 6-year-old Grady was quite perfectionistic and eager to please adults. During this stage he accidentally tossed the bop bag so that it landed on top of a small chair. He grinned, positioned his arms to show off his muscles, and said, "I'm wild!" Children with externalizing problems are likely to engage in more obviously aggressive play, including energetic, competitive, or fighting play. Children with complex trauma and attachment problems often play in intensely aggressive or angry ways. As long as such children do not violate any of the playroom limits, the therapist accepts the aggressive play and the feelings behind it, such as the anger, rage, fear, frustration, or the need for power or control. This is part of the therapeutic process. The therapist's empathic acceptance at the deepest level of feeling helps children move eventually, in their own way and own time, to the next stage.

Regressive Stage

Aggressive behaviors eventually begin to abate, and they are sometimes replaced by a more regressive style of play. Here children may pretend that they are babies, sometimes sucking a baby bottle or asking the therapist to play a parent role with them. Play themes related to attachment and nurturance are common, with the children providing the nurturance, asking for it, or both. Children with strong attachment needs sometimes replay a sequence of development, such as being born, crawling on hands and knees, saying "goo-goo, gaa-gaa," taking tentative first steps, and eventually playing in ways typical of their chronological age. Themes of threat and danger are followed by safety and attachment play. Bad guys threaten, and a child and therapist eventually overcome them.

Mastery Stage

As regressive play themes fade, they give way to themes reflecting various types of mastery: improved problem solving, increased competence, and mastery of fears/anxieties/traumas. The play may reflect the victory of armies or heroes, and children show less evidence of aggressive, fearful, anxious, or regressive play. Children typically show pride in their abilities and accomplishments, whether they are drawing, using a hula hoop, or building a miniature city. Children who previously created their own rules for games to assure that they would beat the therapist are willing to play by the conventional rules at this stage. Problematic behaviors in daily life show considerable improvement during this stage as well.

In general, a therapist can gauge how a child is progressing in therapy by considering the child's passage through these stages. This is not a precise indicator, however, and should only be considered a guide. Other information, such as the child's behavior in daily life and the resolution of the presenting problems, must also be considered.

Levels of Interpretation

Play themes and patterns can be interpreted in different ways. It is useful to consider different levels of interpretation of children's play. O'Connor (2000) has explored five levels of interpretation, and the discussion that follows is loosely based on his work. In CCPT it is useful to consider six levels of interpretation, with successive levels requiring greater therapist reflection and input, due to the uncertainty of knowing another's perceptions and internal realities. Some of these levels are used in CCPT directly with children, while others are used only for therapists' postsession understanding. The six levels are briefly described below.

- *Content.* This refers to a child's overt behaviors and activities. Describing these requires very little therapist interpretation.
- *Feeling.* This refers to the child's emotional expression. Describing this requires a small degree of therapist interpretation, which is accomplished by reading nonverbal cues, facial expressions, and voice intonations. Because most primary emotions are expressed in similar ways by all humans (Ekman, 2007; McConnell, 2006), therapists can be reasonably certain about their readings of the major emotions expressed through children's play. There is greater uncertainty in accurately understanding subtler emotions or degrees of feelings, as these differ culturally and sometimes from family to family.
- *Intention.* This refers to the child's purpose in engaging in a play sequence. Greater therapist interpretation is needed to observe the patterns of play and discern what the child's unstated objectives, plans, or intentions are. Intentions usually cannot be gleaned accurately from single play behaviors.
- *Psychological meaning.* This refers to deeper motivations and explanations of play in terms of psychological theory. An interpretation at this level aims to explain *why* the child plays in a particular way (i.e., what psychological forces are at work or what intrapsychic meaning the play holds). The therapist considers that the play happens *because* of some internal state or process, such as "Betsy keeps rearranging the doll furniture because she is anxious."
- *Relationship of the play to prior sessions.* This refers to ways in which the play in one session is connected to that of previous sessions. This session-to-session pattern provides clues to therapists about the meanings and meaningfulness of the play for children. Sometimes session similarities are quite obvious, and at other times they are so rooted in metaphor that therapists' interpretations are less certain. Session-to-session play can represent themes such as power and control (see "Common Play Themes" below), even though the play activities themselves are quite different in each session.
- *Relationship of the play to daily life or events.* This refers to the ways in which children's play may reflect actual events or situations that have

occurred in their lives, outside the play sessions. Again, the relationship between the play and actual life situations can sometimes be obvious, such as when a child has imaginary car crashes after being in an actual car accident. At other times, the relationship is less obvious; it may be hidden within metaphors that require substantial therapist interpretation, or may remain uncertain without further input.

While any CCPT session is in progress, therapists use only the first three levels of interpretation with children: content, feeling, and intention. In the CCPT environment, if therapists were to comment to children on any of the latter three levels of interpretation, it would tend to interrupt their imaginary play and perhaps stop their play entirely. The first three levels promote an atmosphere of safety, acceptance, and nondirectiveness; the last three are in contrast to such a climate, as they introduce the therapists' own thoughts, judgments, and directions.

Interpretations are used differently in some other forms of play therapy, but in CCPT, therapists reserve their own thoughts for consideration after play sessions have ended and in the service of improving their understanding of children's needs and concerns. Because CCPT therapists trust in children's ability to solve problems through the play process in their own unique ways, they do not believe that the cognitive insights represented by the last three levels of interpretation are necessary for the children to overcome problems. Indeed, CCPT therapists actually try to clear their minds of these last three levels *during* sessions, so that they can attend fully to the children's expressions. They are much more likely to use these deeper interpretations *after* the play sessions, when they are reflecting on the children's progress. These types of interpretations can be useful at this time in helping therapists understand within their own theoretical frameworks what is happening and how to assist with other treatment planning if needed.

Understanding Play Themes in Context

A child's play themes during CCPT should always be interpreted within the total context of the child's and family's experiences. "Cookbook" listings of play items or behaviors and what they might mean cannot provide the rich information about the child's life that is essential for accurate understanding of what the play means from the child's perspective. To borrow loosely from Bronfenbrenner's (1979) ecological model of human development, children are embedded within several nested contexts, and their play themes may reflect the influence of any combination or all of these. They include the following.

• *Individual child.* Influences here include the child's temperament, personality, and sensitivities; development on all dimensions; talents; health; past and present experiences; and hopes and dreams.

• *Immediate family.* Influences include marital and sibling relationships; the health of the family's attachment processes; family routines, interactions, and experiences; parents' employment; the family's unique culture; family development factors; and pets or other animals and how they are incorporated into family life.

• *Extended family.* Influences include those of grandparents, aunts and uncles, cousins, and other extended family members, and their relationships with the child and the child's immediate family. Experiences with the extended family can be influential in both positive and negative ways, and shared experiences can be very important. Extended family members can offer support, but can also apply pressure. Regardless of what their influence is, it should be taken seriously.

• *Community.* Influences at this level include the neighborhood environment, friendships, neighbors, peer relations, school, and religious organizations. Both formal and informal activities at this level can be important, including sports organizations (such as baseball or soccer leagues), Scouting programs, youth groups, community centers, pickup ball games with friends, and music or dance lessons.

• *Broader sociopolitical factors.* Influences here include factors such as poverty or prosperity, wars, disasters, crime rates, unemployment, programs for at-risk children, and family support initiatives.

When a therapist interprets the possible meanings of a child's play, it is useful to consider the circumstances of the child's life in these embedded contexts. Much of this information can be obtained during the assessment process, as well as from discussions with parents held regularly during the period the child is involved in CCPT.

Below are listed some contexts and context-related factors or questions that therapists can consider in regard to children's play themes. Not all are applicable at all times, but they provide additional tools for therapists to use when determining possible meanings of children's play. Coupled with knowledge of children's life circumstances and daily events, these issues can be reviewed as therapists develop working hypotheses and alternative explanations for children's play.

Developmental Context

CCPT therapists consider child development on all dimensions, to determine whether the play themes reflect developmental processes at work. A solid knowledge of developmental theories and progressions is vital. What are the primary developmental tasks for children at this age? Are any of these reflected in the play?

Problem Solving

Therapists also think about problems within the playroom and how children overcome them. The problems often are practical ones. Does a child create or face problems within the playroom (e.g., toys that don't work, difficulty finding what he or she wants), and then find ways to solve them? Is there any type of resolution to the dilemmas or struggles the child is facing in his or her play?

Mastery

As suggested earlier, mastery can relate to developmental and problem-solving processes, to the resolution of psychological issues, or to some combination of these. In trauma work, a child often focuses repeatedly on play themes involving danger and victims, and then creates rescue scenarios or ones in which the child feels powerful, thereby overcoming the foes or the scary feelings. In other instances of repetitive play, where the child seems to be focused on developing a skill (e.g., hitting a target, pouring water into containers), this might suggest developmental mastery—working on eye–hand coordination and so on. Or does the child find play solutions to play dilemmas or to social and emotional dilemmas, even if it's done entirely within the play metaphor? This might show mastery of fears or other emotional or social concerns. For example, if a child plays something about a scary, dangerous dragon, and then finds a way to take away the dragon's powers (magic spell, killing, even more powerful dragon), this might suggest mastery over the fear. Similarly, if a child initially is afraid of a puppet and asks the therapist to put it out of sight for several sessions, then eventually takes it out and plays with it, this suggests that the child is mastering the fear of the puppet by taking control of it.

Family Context

Sometimes children's play reflects their perceptions of family life, roles, feelings, and experiences. What is going on within the family in terms of events or dynamics? Does the play seem related, at least in a general way, to that? For example, if a child plays with a truck so that it goes out of control and crashes into things, does this reflect something about the child's feelings' being out of control, or family relationships' being very conflictual and seemingly out of control? If the child plays with the baby doll a lot, is there a new baby in the family? Is the child experiencing some sibling rivalry with a younger child?

Historical Context

"Historical context" can refer to the child's life history, or to the play history of previous sessions. How might the child's play be reflecting themes or motivations associated with either the recent or more distant past? For example, a child who always plays the figure in control, the boss, or the powerful bad guy may be showing how out of control or victimized he or she felt during past abuse episodes.

Cultural Context

Children's play is universal; it happens in all countries and settings the world over. Their play is embedded within their cultural context and reflects family culture as well as the broader culture. Their play is often reflective of cultural beliefs, practices, symbols, and rituals. Does a child's play reflect cultural symbols? Is it related to culturally relevant beliefs, practices, and experiences? Does the play reflect situations related to racial identity or racism, for example? Does it mimic cultural rituals such as those associated with festivals and holidays, or ceremonies such as weddings or funerals? One of the many reasons why parents are important partners in CCPT is that they may provide important cultural, religious, and other contextual information.

Emotional Tone

"Emotional tone," as noted earlier, refers to the general affective sense the child brings to the play. What's the overall emotional tone of the child's play? What does the child seem to be experiencing? How does the play make the therapist feel? Might the therapist's reactions reveal something about how the child feels in daily life? Is the child playing a role that's the opposite of the role he or she plays in daily life?

What's behind Aggressive Play?

Aggressive play does not necessarily reflect anger or violence, although it can. It is important to distinguish between aggressive *play* and *actual* violent or destructive behavior. The motivations and dynamics behind these can be quite different. What is the aggressive play *really* communicating or doing for the child? For example, does it make the child feel more in control or powerful? Does it help the child feel less like a victim and more like a victor? Does it reflect perseverance over obstacles? Does it help the child build a sense of self-efficacy? Adults sometimes react too strongly to the surface appearance of children's play, interpreting it literally without exploring what it means to the children themselves. This is especially true of confusing feelings such as anger, or behaviors such as aggressive play. Almost always there are more fundamental feelings beneath the anger or aggression, and these should be the focus of understanding. (Suggested resources for understanding children's aggressive play include L. F. Guerney, 2001; Jones, 2002; and Mechling, 2008.)

The Good and the Bad of It

Most personal characteristics have both a good and a bad side, depending on the degree to which they are present, and whether they are functional or dysfunctional. A child whose play is quite obsessive may also be quite organized or planful. A child who changes play frequently may also be spontaneous and imaginative. A child who worries excessively about what others think of his or her play may also be sensitive and caring. Therapists should consider the dual nature of many characteristics. Hidden within the problems lie strengths that can help moderate children's reactions or behaviors in healthier, more balanced directions. For example, an anxious child who always worries about getting things right may eventually relax a bit during play sessions to a point where he or she can tolerate making some mistakes or messes; yet the child is likely to retain the desire to do a good job. In fact, the play sessions can provide the nonjudgmental atmosphere needed for the child to practice making mistakes in order to dissipate his or her anxiety about this.

This listing of contexts and context-related issues in children's play should not be considered exhaustive, but it may provide some guidance for therapists as they consider each session's play themes and potential meanings.

Common Play Themes

Because children's play in CCPT is embedded within the various contexts of their lives, there are thousands of interpretations that can be made. Some common play themes include the following:

- Power and control
- Aggression
- Different emotions, including joy, sadness, anger, and fear
- Good versus evil
- Winning and losing
- Mastery of developmental tasks
- Mastery of fears or anxiety
- Trauma reenactment and mastery
- Identity
- Boundaries
- Grief and loss
- Nurturance
- Regression
- Attachment
- Danger/threat, usually coupled with safety/rescue/protection
- Resilience
- Persistence
- Problem solving
- Cultural symbols, customs, and rituals
- Desires and wishes

Suggestions about the Interpretation of Play Themes

Therapists' interpretations of children's play themes in CCPT are necessarily influenced by the therapists' preferred theoretical orientations. Because the deeper-level interpretations are not shared directly with children, it poses no problem if therapists see some play themes differently from their colleagues. A psychodynamically oriented therapist and a behaviorally oriented therapist are likely to think about children's play very differently. In order to stay within the child's frame of reference as well as the humanistic principles underlying CCPT, however, it is important to remember that the most important interpretation is the child's own. The play means something to the child in that particular time and place, and the key is to seek an accurate understanding from this point of view rather than to "analyze" the child.

There are many times when a therapist simply does not understand what the play means to a child or cannot interpret it in any of the contexts of which the therapist may be aware. This is not a problem. Once again, the key is to stay attuned to the expressions and feelings of the child in the playroom, and to accept with humility that therapists cannot always figure things out. A fundamental assumption that when an atmosphere of safety and acceptance is created, children will play and grow in a healthy direction, helps CCPT therapists *trust the process*!

Finally, it is essential for a therapist who is first learning CCPT to obtain supervision from an experienced nondirective play therapy professional. Not only can this help with skill development in a wide array of circumstances, but it can develop the therapist's ability to remain focused on the child while attempting to understand the play themes within a contextual framework.

Documentation of Themes and Progress

Like all child therapists, play therapists document their sessions in some form of progress notes. Sometimes therapists who use CCPT wonder how this is done when the therapy revolves around child-directed play.

As we discuss in greater detail in Chapter 7, therapists create a treatment plan based on the parents' descriptions of the presenting problems, coupled with information gleaned in the assessment process. Specific therapeutic goals can be set in behavioral language (i.e., in terms that can be quantifiably measured). Common goals for CCPT include reduction or elimination of the presenting problems, such as a reduction in the number and frequency of sibling arguments, or the elimination of biting and hitting behaviors. Often CCPT therapists include as goals the development or improvement of problem-solving skills, or the achievement of mastery over a fear or situation. These typically happen in the course of CCPT and lead to better overall functioning. Other goals, such as decreased parental stress, can be included as well. These goals are then used as key markers to determine whether progress is being made.

It may not be obvious to professionals without training and experience in CCPT how children's play session behaviors relate to the goals listed on their treatment plans. It is valuable for a therapist to document sessions in a way that helps draw the connections between what happens in the sessions and the goals, thereby making it clearer whether or not a child is progressing. To do this, a three-part progress note, typically one to two pages long, is useful.

The first section briefly describes the child's actual behaviors in the play session. This need not be detailed. For example, the note might read:

> Amanda moved around the playroom quickly at first, looking at and touching many of the toys. After 5 minutes, she sat by the dollhouse and arranged and rearranged furniture for 10 minutes. She played by herself with the puppets, concentrating on the cat and kitten puppets, who were "hanging around in the barn." During the final 5 minutes, she drew a house and garden on the whiteboard, with a smiling mother, daughter, and baby by the front door.

The second section discusses the therapist's tentative interpretations, or possible play themes. Applying the concepts presented in this chapter, the therapist records play themes that seem to fit the child's play, given his or her contextual knowledge of the child. For instance, the therapist might write:

> Amanda initially explored the playroom, then played several family-related themes. She seemed interested in how the various family characters related to each other. She focused on families who were happy together.

The third section ties the therapist's observations and interpretations back to the goals established for the child. This should be done tentatively unless the therapist is certain of the connection. Furthermore, there may be some sessions during which the connection is not clear, and the therapist can wait until future sessions provide more information before recording any connections. To continue the example of Amanda, her therapist might write:

Amanda seems to be working on family relationships, exploring how people relate to each other in happy ways. This is in stark contrast to her experiences with her biological family, but it seems to indicate an interest in relationships and her desire to establish closer family ties. It appears that she is working on issues relating to achieving a healthier attachment with less discord (i.e., Goal 3, reducing conflict and arguments with her foster mother). Her foster mother also reported that Amanda has been asking her to read to her at bedtime. This also demonstrates progress on Goal 3.

This is one way to help educate anyone who may read the documentation about the child's progress. Some agencies may have a different method for documenting sessions, but the basic ideas here can still be applied. The key is to avoid overstepping or overinterpreting information. In many cases, parent reports of behaviors at home are useful to include as well. Again, supervision is important for therapists without much experience in documentation of therapy sessions, as there are many legal and ethical matters involved.

PART III

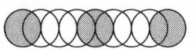

PARENT INVOLVEMENT

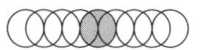

CHAPTER 7

Engaging Parents (and Teachers) in Child-Centered Play Therapy

Parents, after struggling with emotional or behavioral problems with their children, often wish and believe that child therapists will know just the right words to say and things to do that will somehow change the children's behavior. CCPT therapists frequently must explain to parents that no one can talk someone else out of their problems, including children. Often one of therapists' first tasks during initial meetings with parents is to educate them about child development and child play in a manner that engages them in the therapeutic process, even though it bears little resemblance to their expectations. Some thoughts that therapists can share with parents follow.

During childhood, most of what children learn is through play. Play is a child's preferred mode of expression. Play is also a metaphor for the conscious and unconscious material that the child has not yet learned how to put into words. Therefore, play is the vehicle by which CCPT explores the unconscious world of the child.

Children are not miniature adults. They are young people with minimal life experiences and not fully developed brains who face the tremendous tasks of learning about themselves, the world in which they

live, and the best ways to cope in that huge world. Although the learning required of children is monumental, children have innate abilities
and enormous brain capacity to master what they need to know to function in a healthy way in a complex world. CCPT therapists, who are well
grounded in the stages of child development, have learned to appreciate
children's abilities to master themselves and to solve their own problems when placed in an environment of understanding, acceptance,
and safety. That environment is the CCPT playroom accompanied by a
fully trained CCPT therapist.

Introducing Parents to CCPT:
The Importance of Empathy

When parents seek treatment for their children, they come fully armed
with questions, defensiveness, and feelings of inadequacy. Even though
most have never been taught good parenting skills, parents know that
society bases its judgment of their performance as parents on how their
children present themselves in the real world. Child therapists must
adopt a nonjudgmental stance when interacting with parents. Parents
are not given a manual on how to raise a child or be good parents when
a child is born. Most adults are given far more information and instructions about a new car or gadget than about the most complex task they
are likely to face in their lives—raising a child. The huge majority of
parents *want* to be good parents; they just may not know how.

   With this in mind, CCPT therapists must join with parents in the
quest to help their children. Parents are neither their children's enemies
nor the therapists'. In fact, parents are valuable members of the treatment team. Parents can provide great insight into their children and
family lives. They are the ones who live with their children 24 hours
a day, 7 days a week—observing, knowing, and loving the children.
As such, parents have a wealth of knowledge about their children that
will help the therapeutic process. Therapists need to let parents know
that they value their input, continuing observations, and involvement
in the process. This collaborative approach is much more likely to yield
success.

   Before a therapist recommends or starts CCPT with a child, an
intake meeting with just the parents can provide the therapist with valuable information. During that session, the most important thing is for
the therapist to listen empathically to the parents' concerns. Empathic

listening about, and genuine acceptance of, the parents' feelings and concerns will set the tone for the parents to begin trusting the therapist. Only after parents feel that their concerns have been heard and their own feelings understood will they be able to entrust their child to the therapist. Moreover, a therapist who hears parents' concerns thoroughly and well is in a much better position to provide meaningful rationales to parents for the CCPT approach. For example, imagine giving the parents of an oppositional child the opportunity to vent their frustration as to how "nothing works" when it comes to disciplining their child. This information opens a door for the therapist. The parents have talked; they have been heard; and now they are ready to hear what the therapist has to say. At this point, the therapist can explain how when discipline does not work, it is because there are underlying unresolved feelings that the child acts out because the child does not know how to express those feelings any other way. The therapist can continue by saying,

> Play is a child's primary means of expression. Children will find appropriate ways to vent these unresolved feelings in play therapy so that they won't have to act them out. Also, as part of the play therapy process, children learn that they are responsible for their own behavior. This allows them to learn internal controls, which enable them to recognize that their choices result in consequences. That is, if their behavior is within appropriate limits, the consequence is a positive one. If the behavior goes beyond the limits, the consequence is a negative one."

Quite often parents worry about their child's self-esteem. They may relate how teachers react punitively to their child or how peers are rejecting. Again, after listening empathically and well, the therapist will have an opportunity to speak about the principles of CCPT. This explanation can include how play therapy allows children to master themselves, their own feelings, and their behavior, and how this mastery results in improved self-esteem. The therapist can go on to explain how each negative event in a child's life can put a dent in the child's self-esteem. Thus, when a child is scolded by an adult, struggles in school, or is made fun of by a peer, all of these dents add up to major self-esteem damage. When children learn through play therapy that they have control over the consequences of their own actions, they begin to make better choices with positive results, and ultimately develop increased self-worth.

As these examples illustrate, a therapist who listens well can tie the recommendations for CCPT or any other intervention directly to the parents' concerns. When the therapist helps the parents understand the connections between their child's problems and the CCPT process, the parents are able to appreciate how the play therapy approach is exactly what is needed to help their child.

Establishing Treatment Goals

Before establishing treatment goals, the therapist will find it valuable to invite the parents, the child identified with the presenting problem, and any siblings living in the home to participate in a family play observation. The entire family plays in the playroom while the therapist observes for 15–20 minutes. This process helps the therapist get a sense of the target child's behavior and of how that child relates to other members of the family. This understanding of the child in the context of the family system is important for any form of child intervention.

During the family play observation, the therapist sits unobtrusively in a corner of the room, just outside the open door to the playroom, or in an observation booth if one is available. The therapist tells the family to play and have fun, as if the therapist is not there. The therapist pays attention to the interactions among family members; methods used by the parents to control the children's behavior; problematic behaviors or interactions; and any signs of neurological or biological problems (hyperactivity, distractibility, speech problems, awkward gait, tics, hearing issues, etc.). The therapist is interested in learning about the quality of attachments, boundaries, parenting styles, family roles, and communication processes. At the end of the observation, the therapist meets with only the parents and asks them how similar or dissimilar the playtime was to home interactions. After empathically listening to their reactions, the play therapist summarizes his or her observations. The therapist also explores with parents any concerns that might be outside the scope of CCPT but that warrant a referral or continuing awareness, such as speech or neurological problems.

Beyond providing the play therapist with valuable information, the family play observation session is a good way to introduce the child and parents to the special room (the playroom) and the play materials that will be used in CCPT. After the observation, it is important to ask parents whether they have any questions or concerns about the playroom or the toys with which the child will be playing. This gives the play therapist an opportunity to address any concerns the parents may have about dart guns, aggression toys, or any other toys they might consider inappropriate for their child. Once again, the play therapist needs to be sensitive to the parents' feelings by responding empathically to their concerns. After the parents feel fully heard, it is then appropriate to provide rationales for the inclusion of various toys, or perhaps to decide to include other toys at the parents' request. For example, if parents remark that the toys are too "babyish" for their child, the therapist might consider adding a toy or two that the parents think may benefit their child, as long as these meet the criteria for good playroom toys. Usually, however, listening to the parents' concerns and providing rationales are sufficient in these instances. Furthermore, simply because a parent has concerns about certain toys does not mean that these toys should automatically be removed from or included in the playroom. It is prudent, however, to discuss the matter fully with the parents, so that they understand and accept the final decisions about the toys.

When the therapist is meeting with parents to begin the process of CCPT, it is important to establish a beneficial team relationship with them by including them in the development of treatment goals. It would be appropriate to ask the parents such questions as these: "What are your goals for your child's treatment?", "What types of changes are you expecting from treatment?", "Does your child have difficulty expressing feelings appropriately?", "Do you have concerns about your child's self-esteem?", "What are some of the issues the school has identified?", and/or "Do you have concerns about how you and your spouse handle discipline?" Based on the information parents provide, the play therapist records specific goals for treatment and shares them with the parents, so that the collaborative relationship is maintained.

Handling Parental Resistance

Although parents bring their children to treatment, the parents themselves may feel threatened by the process. Some parents feel coerced by well-meaning pediatricians or school personnel to seek treatment for their children. Parents who feel inadequate may worry that the play therapist will win the affections of their children, casting the parents into a secondary position in the children's lives. Yet other parents may worry that the children or their treatment will reveal their inadequacies as parents.

Unless play therapists remain sensitive to these feelings and the issues underlying them, parents may unwittingly (or even knowingly) sabotage the play therapy. An example of near-sabotage occurred when a mother insisted that her 6-year-old son needed treatment as the result of marital discord between the parents. Although both parents generally brought their son to treatment, the father clearly was not thrilled about the process. Sensing the father's displeasure with therapy, the son was extremely reluctant to express himself openly in play therapy. When the play therapist empathically acknowledged the father's apparent displeasure, he admitted that he was not a fan of therapy because his very troubled sister had responded poorly in therapy as a child; once she became an adult, she had abandoned her family. Once the therapist accepted and acknowledged his fears, this father was able to recognize that his experience with his sister did not mean that his son's involvement in therapy would result in the same outcome. Ultimately the father was able to start engaging in the play therapy process, and he even began to recognize how his anger toward his son about the son's negative behavior was not productive. With the help of the play therapist, the father eventually learned to set more appropriate limits with his son, thereby diminishing the father's anger and improving the son's behavior.

When parents insist that they want their children in talk therapy, not play therapy, there may be some other barriers to overcome. Being sensitive to the parents' concerns and listening empathically are the keys to working through this dilemma. Once therapists understand parents' concerns, they are in a better position to provide a rationale for their treatment of choice, and the parents are in a better place to hear what therapists are recommending. For example, Randy, a 7-year-old boy, was referred for treatment. He was a child with extremely high intelligence who was brought to therapy by two equally bright parents. Randy was very immature both socially and emotionally, however. His parents thought that he was an ideal candidate for talk therapy, and regarded play therapy as too "babyish" for a child of his intellect. Although the parents initially agreed to follow the play therapist's recommendations for CCPT, they quickly became dissatisfied with Randy's progress in treatment. At the parents' insistence, the play therapist agreed to introduce some more directive approaches as part of the therapy hour to help Randy achieve his treatment goals.

After two brief sessions of talk therapy and the use of some role-playing techniques to help Randy interact with peers more appropriately, it became evident that Randy was not interested in anything except going into the special room—where he was fully engaged and used a great deal of play to address the issues of his rejection by peers, his feeling that he was a "weird kid," and his fantasy of being a special child with unique powers. When given the choice of going into the "talking room" or the special room, Randy always chose the latter, much to the parents' dismay. What became clear to the play therapist was that Randy's parents did not really like the child he was and wanted someone to make him into someone they could like. When this issue was addressed with the parents (with the appropriate sensitivity), the father acknowledged that he himself had always been the weird though bright child in school, and he could not stand to watch his son go through what he did as a child. Also, the mother admitted that her husband had no real friends except for the social connections she had made for them as a couple, and she didn't want her son to grow up to be unhappy like his father. Ultimately it was determined that the father would probably benefit from treatment of his own, though there was a tremendous amount of resistance to starting that process. Randy continued in CCPT until the family left for their summer shore home, though the parents agreed that they would have Randy resume CCPT in the fall, as well as sign him up for a social skills group. It should be noted that Randy's progress in CCPT at the time of this writing has been slow, and his prognosis is guarded. The therapist hopes, however, that the restart of CCPT during the next school year in conjunction with a social skills group will be a good combination to help the parents get more "on board" with the treatment plan.

Resistance to treatment is a complicated matter. Elsewhere, VanFleet (2000b, 2007) has explored the causes of parental resistance to play therapy in some detail, and has offered effective approaches for engaging parents more fully. In general, CCPT therapists must make every effort to "stay the course" while helping parents navigate the issues involved in their resistance to recommendations for their child's treatment. Showing sensitivity to parental concerns, listening empathically, and working as a team with parents offer the best chance for helping parents accept the validity of play therapy. Sometimes therapists just need to remind parents to be patient with the process. Although CCPT often results in rapid changes in children, this is not always the case. Children and their families are complex systems. It can be helpful to remind parents that children's problems do not pop up overnight, and that the process of change cannot be hurried to make problems go away quickly. (As we discuss in a later chapter, it is sometimes possible to augment CCPT with more directive play or family interventions, as long as they do not interfere with CCPT. These should not be implemented with the idea that they will speed up the therapeutic process, however.)

If parents insist on finding a "quick fix," they may become frustrated and end CCPT prematurely or seek help elsewhere. Although empathy and patience will help therapists engage most parents in the process, sometimes parental resistance cannot be overcome. In these cases, it is important for therapists to learn from the situation as best they can, and then to focus on the successes they have experienced in CCPT.

Regular Meetings with Parents

When therapists decide to work with children, they need to be prepared to work with parents. Certainly it is helpful to have some familiarity with family systems theory and family therapy (Ginsberg, 1997; Minuchin, 1974; Sori, 2006). Excellent CCPT can only be enhanced by parental involvement; conversely, it can be undermined by parents who unwittingly sabotage the process (as described above), or who contribute to a child's ongoing problems through poor parenting skills. Child therapists need to determine the extent of possible parental involvement in each case, but they should recognize that parents always need to be involved to some degree, even if it's simply to touch base to discuss their children's progress. Because parents have sought therapy, it is likely that they are eager for assistance and motivated for change, even though they may not be expecting what therapists suggest.

For parents who demonstrate or verbalize difficulties with limit setting, their involvement in the therapeutic process should be significant. Without good limit setting in the home environment, children's issues may never be resolved or may require an extensive course of treatment before the children learn internal controls. Structure and clear limits create the safety children need to express themselves and to grow and develop in healthy ways. Families with serious difficulties in establishing structure or limits at home may require two sessions per week—one for the CCPT, and another for educating and monitoring parents with limit setting at home. Once the parents acquire and maintain limit-setting skills, the second weekly session can be eliminated; however, it is recommended that 10–15 minutes of a child's therapy hour be devoted to a check-in regarding the parents' continued progress.

Sometimes parents fear that if they set limits their children won't like them, but the opposite is true: Children thrive when limits are clear, because they feel more secure when they know their parents are in charge. They may not like a specific limit, but the more general impact is an enhanced sense of security. If parents waver when they tell children "no," it may be difficult for children to believe anything they say, even "I love you." Often parents have not viewed their dynamics this way.

An example where a child's therapy was undermined by one parent's failure to set clear and consistent limits and consequences involved a 6-year-old boy named Dane. His mother was a pediatrician who worked long hours, and his father was a stay-at-home dad. The father was an anxious and fearful man who tended to be overprotective, and he resorted to yelling as a means to control his son. The son was also highly anxious, and repeatedly told his mother that he felt unloved and wanted to kill himself. The mother also failed to follow through with appropriate limits and consequences because she could not get her husband to unite with her in her efforts. The father was a challenge because he had had a very difficult childhood fraught with illnesses and parents who were not good role models for him. Many sessions were spent with the parents in discussing the rationale for limits and consequences, and in trying to help them develop and implement these skills at home. Dane even told the therapist during his CCPT sessions that he was in treatment because of his father. The therapist held some individual sessions with the father, to better understand his history and to help him connect his own life experiences to his difficulties in setting appropriate limits with his son. With much patience and empathic listening from the therapist, the father eventually came to understand that his failure to set appropriate limits was undermining his son's progress. Eventually, and with consistent reinforcement of the father's efforts, the therapist helped the parents to formulate a plan for better limits and structure at home; this in turn helped Dane progress in his CCPT sessions. Because of the many hurdles involved, it required a year of intensive work with the father individually and the parents together for them to achieve consistency in the implementation of their plan.

In situations where parents have relatively good parenting skills, and the child is in therapy for issues arising from parental divorce, death of a family member, difficult peer relationships, or learning problems, parental involvement may be less intensive. In such cases, approximately 10 minutes of a child's therapy hour can be devoted to updating the parents on the child's play themes, monitoring the child's progress through reports of home and school behavior changes, answering parents' questions, or helping the parents with some minor issues they are encountering with the child in the home. Therapists also sometimes help parents with other home interventions, such as establishing good bedtime routines, creating behavior modification programs for chores or morning routines, structuring an environment conducive to doing homework, and so on. Sometimes during these regular parent meetings, it becomes apparent that a school meeting may be needed to address issues related to the child's school behavior or learning.

Long-term CCPT can support children if they live with highly dysfunctional parents who do not have the capacity to change their parenting, or if they are involved in the child protective and/or foster care system. For example, Louise Guerney treated a mother who was extremely narcissistic and dependent. The father, though less self-centered, was poorly educated and inadequate. They had two children, and their son was extremely hyperactive. After the intake assessments, Dr. Guerney believed that the high level of individual dysfunction in the parents precluded them from being good candidates for FT. As she worked with the mother individually, Dr. Guerney found one graduate student after another to work with the hyperactive son, Stephen (with each student typically working with the boy for a year). Stephen avidly went to the play sessions each week for years. He played hard and used every session to vent his energy, frustration, anger, and other feelings. Occasionally Stephen missed a week of therapy; inevitably, Dr. Guerney would later receive a phone call from the school principal wondering whether Stephen was still involved in play therapy. The answer was always "yes," as Dr. Guerney knew that his would be a long-term case, and the principal was always relieved to hear her answer. Stephen's ongoing involvement in CCPT was the "glue" he needed to hold himself together in school each week, despite his highly dysfunctional parents.

Handling Behavior Issues

Much of CCPT therapists' consultation work with parents aims to help them use more effective parenting skills in the home environment. This is often accomplished through the use of "teachable moments." When parents ask for advice on handling home behavior issues, therapists have an opportunity to teach them how to use skills at home that closely resemble those used by therapists in CCPT sessions, such as structuring, limit setting, and empathic listening. All of these skills can be broken down into teachable parts and covered with parents across several consultations. The book *Parenting: A Skills Training Manual* (L. F. Guerney, 1995) is an excellent resource for doing this. Therapists can also help parents understand the theory and implementation of good behavioral reinforcement programs. Sometimes it becomes obvious that parents would also benefit from their own individual treatment or marital/couple counseling. When this arises, therapists must be sensitive to the parents' feelings and reactions, while making a referral to another therapist in whom they have confidence.

Frequently parents have concerns about controlling their children's behavior not only at home, but in public. There is nothing more embarrassing for parents than to have their children act up in a public place, and nothing more frustrating than a child who will not listen to them. When parents raise questions about controlling behavior, therapists can share how limits are handled in CCPT via the three-step procedure of stating the rule, giving a warning, and implementing the consequence. It is also helpful for parents to understand how to establish appropriate consequences for negative behavior, including natural, related, and unrelated consequences. Therapists can help parents understand these concepts and how to apply them to the problems they describe.

"Natural consequences" are naturally occurring results of negative behavior. Examples of such consequences include being laughed at by other children for nose picking or the like, skinning one's knee when running on a slippery pool surface, or burning one's hand when touching a hot stove. When natural consequences occur, parents do not need to intervene. The natural process provides the corrective feedback children need to recognize that their negative behavior results in negative consequences. Of course, parents cannot always allow natural consequences to occur, because some consequences would be too severe. The natural consequence of running into the street is getting hit by a car, and that simply is not an option for parents to allow! In cases where natural consequences are dangerous or do not suffice, parents must intervene with other types of consequences.

The most useful parent-imposed consequence is called a "related consequence." Related consequences mean that "the punishment fits the crime," or that the consequences are related in some way to the misbehavior. For example, if a child won't sit in his or her chair at dinner, a parent sends the child out of the room for 5 minutes, away from the family meal. This shows children that if they want to be with the family during meals, they must sit in their chairs. If two children are fighting over a toy, a parent imposes a related consequence by taking the toy away from both of them for a short period of time. Time out is considered a related consequence if it is used for attention-getting behavior, such as acting up in a store to get a toy, walking in front of the television to annoy a sibling, or fighting with a sibling to get a parent's attention while the parent is on the telephone. Related consequences are generally quite effective, as the consequences are meaningful to a child.

"Unrelated consequences" have no direct connection to the negative behavior. Examples of unrelated consequences include loss of television privileges for fighting with a sibling, loss of computer access for not cleaning up one's room, or not being allowed to play outside with friends because of talking back to a parent. Natural and related consequences work better, but if parents cannot think of a related consequence, unrelated consequences will do.

Therapists also must help parents understand that harshness or severity of a consequence is not what changes children's behaviors, and that severe methods often have the opposite effect of what parents might expect. When consequences are overly harsh, or are delivered in an angry manner, children are likely to forget the reason they are being punished and to focus on their anger and resentment at their parents for being so unfair. The word "discipline" comes from a Latin word meaning "to teach," not "to punish." Children learn best when the consequence is meaningful, related in some way to the negative behavior, and consistently enforced once a warning has been given.

Therapists can help parents understand that yelling and spanking are never good or effective consequences. Generally these parental reactions occur because a parent has waited too long to give a warning and/or to implement an appropriate consequence. Yelling is often interpreted by children as a reward; they actually enjoy hearing parents lose their tempers, because this suggests that the parents have lost control. Many children secretly enjoy the power they have to bring their parents to this point.

It can be helpful to explain to parents that all behavior has consequences, and that good parenting requires making sure children get appropriate positive or negative consequences for their behavior. Very often, parents are reinforcing negative behavior without realizing it. For example, if the parent pays attention to a child who is seeking attention in a negative way, the parent is actually rewarding the negative behavior. If 3-year-old Angie is having a temper tantrum because her mother is not letting her sit on her lap during dinner, her mother will be rewarding or reinforcing temper tantrums if she picks Angie up to comfort her. Although the mother's behavior may stop the temper tantrum at that moment, the mother is setting herself up for bigger and better temper tantrums when Angie does not get her own way the next time.

In a society where children have learned to expect instant gratification because they get all of the material things they want, parents often have difficulty finding rewards for appropriate behavior. Therapists can help parents learn that the best reward for children is to receive their parents' undivided attention for appropriate behavior. Some time ago, a therapist worked with a mother who had a great deal of difficulty getting her 6-year-old son, Charlie, out of bed and ready for school. The mother decided to try a reward program and told Charlie that if he was completely ready for school by 8:20 A.M., he could watch 20 minutes of television before heading out to the bus stop. For the first week, Charlie was up and ready for school at the agreed-upon time, and earned his 20 minutes of TV. By the second week, Charlie was not as interested in watching TV, so he started giving his mother a hard time again. It was clear from what the mother described that Charlie was being resistant about getting ready for school because he liked the attention (albeit negative) that he received from his mother. Once this was explained to the mother, she decided to offer Charlie 20 minutes of playing a game or doing some other fun activity with her if he was ready on time without a fuss. Charlie immediately began cooperating again with the reinforcement program and earning his 20 minutes of playtime, with his mother giving him her undivided attention. By the end of the first week, Charlie asked his mother to go outside with him, sit on the curb together, and wait for the bus. As they sat on the curb discussing the upcoming day, Charlie spotted a caterpillar crossing the road. Charlie and his mother watched the caterpillar until the bus arrived. Much to his mother's surprise, Charlie grabbed his mother, gave her a big hug, and told her it was the best morning he'd ever had. This mother's gift of her complete attention to Charlie during this otherwise boring activity, and Charlie's positive reaction, make a case in point for the value of parental attention as a superior reward for children's positive behavior.

Therapists can also suggest that parents reserve items they might normally purchase for their children as rewards for good behavior. If a child is accustomed to getting a small toy whenever he or she goes shopping with a parent, the parent can use the trinket as a reward for good behavior (staying by the parent's side in the store, not whining while the parent is shopping, etc.). Of course, if the child does not comply with the expected behavior, it is equally important for the parent to with-hold the toy so as not to reward negative behavior. These suggestions may seem simplistic to our readers, but some parents do not understand how they inadvertently reinforce misbehavior, nor do they know how to turn it around. By helping parents learn to do this more effectively in everyday situations, therapists are teaching them how to use positive and negative consequences in ways that teach children what is expected of them.

Preventing Behavior Problems

Structuring is another useful skill therapists can help parents apply at home. For example, time warnings can be extremely effective in getting cooperative behavior from children. Consider how badly adults would react if someone came into the room while they were writing an e-mail, pulled them off their laptops, put their coats on them, and dragged them out to the car. This type of interaction occurs for children in some form or fashion every day. It would take just a little thought and planning to give children a 5-minute warning to end their playtime, get ready to go out, put their coats on, and come out to the car. Therapists can help parents make short time notifications to their children as part of their routines. For example, when parents pick up their children at a friend's house, they can make the transition easier if they arrive early and give the children a 10- or 15-minute notice to wind down their activities. For this to work, however, parents then need to follow through within whatever time frame they establish. Children have good internal time clocks and can learn to ignore time warnings if an adult gives 5-minute warnings, only to make the children wait for 20 minutes.

Other structuring methods may include making job charts, doing a picture chart of a child's morning or evening routine, or preparing the child in advance for a visit to the dentist or for getting a shot at the pediatrician's office. Structuring gives children the support they need to help them cope in a world that has many expectations and is much bigger than they are.

Another form of structuring skill involves prevention of commonly occurring problems. Therapists can explore with parents some of the problems that occur over and over again. The task is to plan ahead in order to avoid the problem completely. For example, if two children come into the house after school and immediately begin squabbling with each other, the key is for the parent to intervene the minute they walk through the door, *before* they begin arguing. In this case, structuring might include having a snack ready as soon as they get home; giving them a cooperative and fun task to do; or asking them to go to their rooms without speaking to each other to change their clothing, and then sitting with the two of them so they can each talk about their day for a few minutes. In essence, the therapist helps parents learn how to identify the antecedent conditions and how to structure the situation so that the usual problem never has a chance to emerge.

Helping Children with Their Feelings

Empathic or reflective listening is another skill from CCPT that can be extremely useful in the home setting. Feelings often drive behavior, and if feelings are not acknowledged, people tend to act feelings out through their behavior. This is not just true for children. Consider a harried working mother whose husband has not been supportive of her efforts to establish better rules and consequences for the children. If she doesn't express her disappointment or frustration to her husband directly, she may act it out by "forgetting" to pick up his dry cleaning or being "too tired" when he wants sexual intimacy. Although adults have much more ability to express feelings and needs than children, they are often timid or lacking in good communication skills to convey their needs. Children are still in the process of learning about their feelings and are likely to have even more difficulty expressing themselves adequately or in appropriate ways. If direct communication is difficult for adults, it is virtually impossible for children who do not understand their feelings well or do not believe that anyone is understanding them.

Parents can learn to use the empathic listening skill at home to help children learn about their feelings. Some parents may need assistance identifying underlying feelings and developing the "language of feelings." Sometimes a list of feeling words can familiarize parents with the vocabulary of emotion. Therapists can also listen to issues parents raise about their children, look for the children's feelings that are underlying the problem or behavior, and suggest ways for parents to respond to their children. An angry child is usually hurt, scared, or frustrated, but all the parent may see is anger. Showing them how to find and respond to the deeper feelings can make a big difference in their parenting. For example, if a father reports that his daughter comes home from school looking dejected, the therapist can encourage the father to identify feelings the child may be having, and can help him put them into an empathic statement. Thus, if the father thinks his daughter looks sad or bothered, he can state to the child, "Something seems to be bothering you," or "You seem very sad right now." The more difficult task is to have the parent wait for the child to respond, rather than jumping in with questions about what is wrong. Parents can be reminded that questions often backfire with children, as they don't know why they feel the way they do or may simply not like being questioned. Also, particularly with parents who think they must solve all of their children's problems, it is important to stress that simply showing understanding of the children's feelings is frequently all that is necessary for the children to move past a problem. Often nothing more needs to be done.

Therapists can also urge parents to pay attention to children's positive feelings and to acknowledge them to the children in empathic statements. It is valuable for parents to understand that truly good self-esteem comes from children's recognition of their own positive feelings. This knowledge helps motivate parents to look for these opportunities. For example, if Susie comes home with a good report card and proudly states, "Look at this!", an excellent response would be "You are so proud of yourself for getting such a good report card." Of course, the parent can still state how proud he or she is of the child, but it is good practice for parents to acknowledge the child's own positive feelings before volunteering their judgment about the child's performance.

It is also helpful for parents to learn that self-esteem depends on children's ability to cope effectively with negative emotions as well. When children are upset and voice self-deprecating thoughts, parents can reflect the feelings of disappointment and frustration before helping the children shift their self-appraisals toward greater realism.

All the skills and interventions with parents discussed so far take time and practice for parents to master. Many parents did not have good role models in their own parents, and they appreciate this type of help and direction. In turn, CCPT therapists should strive to be good models for the parents with whom they work. Very often, children's waiting room behavior gives an opportunity to do this kind of modeling for the parents to witness, and perhaps this modeling can be discussed later with the parents. With this in mind, a therapist should aim always to demonstrate empathy and attunement to feelings, for the children as well as the parents. For example, if a parent rushes into the waiting room with a child, the therapist can acknowledge the hasty arrival: "You seem very harried. It must have been difficult to get here." If the child slumps in a waiting room chair with a long face, the therapist might state, "You seem sad today." The therapist can also model good limit setting by stating to a child who is pulling out a lot of toys in the waiting room before the session, "Remember that I clean up the toys in the playroom, and the rule is that you must clean up the toys in the waiting room before we begin our play session." Therapists have many opportunities to demonstrate the skills of good parenting throughout the CCPT process, both as play therapists and as models for the parents.

To become true experts in working with parents, therapists need continuing professional development to keep abreast of trends in child rearing, common childhood problems, research, and readings for parents. Two excellent sources of information for both therapists and parents are the aforementioned *Parenting: A Skills Training Manual* (L. F. Guerney, 1995) and *Playful Parenting* (Cohen, 2001).

Handling of School Issues

Children are often referred for treatment because their behavioral issues are problematic in the school environment. Like parents, school personnel can be valuable members of the treatment team. Once a referral is made by a school teacher, counselor, or principal, the wise play therapist asks the parent to sign a release-of-information form that will permit communication between the therapist and school personnel. In making the initial contact with the school, the therapist may introduce him- or herself, listen to the school's concerns about the child, and talk about the CCPT approach. The therapist can also offer to consult by phone about the child's problematic school behavior as needed. In some cases, a therapist may observe a child in the school setting and offer suggestions to the teacher or others involved. During work with teachers— who, like parents, can be defensive or mistrustful of an outside therapist—it is important to apply the same principles of empathic listening and acknowledgment of the teachers' role as valuable team members in children's treatment.

Just as therapists work with parents to apply the skills of CCPT to real-life situations, they can do the same with teachers or other school personnel. The sharing of information and impressions can be beneficial to both teachers and therapists. Elementary school teachers spend over 30 hours a week with their students, so therapists should take time to listen to their input before offering suggestions. Empathic listening goes a long way with educators, just as it does with parents. Even in cases where the teachers may be contributing to the problem, it is advisable to engage them in the process by using the same relationship-building skills discussed earlier for use with parents.

For their part, therapists might discuss themes in the children's play and the children's reactions to limit setting, while helping teachers assess the most effective ways to handle the children's behavior in the classroom and other school environments. Therapists should also prepare teachers for possible changes in children's behavior during the treatment process, including the possibility of negative school behaviors when the children enter an angry stage in treatment. Continued collaboration can yield practical steps teachers can take to handle troublesome behaviors that emerge during the therapy process.

In-school observations typically occur with the goal of establishing a behavior plan to help children demonstrate more self-control in the classroom, in the lunchroom, or during recess. Once a behavioral program is established, therapists are well advised to invite teachers to contact them with any implementation questions or concerns, and to follow up within a few days to a week to see how things are going. Whenever possible, it is also helpful to have teachers track the children's behavior on a simple chart. It is also important to warn teachers that behaviors sometimes get worse before improving.

One such school observation was particularly interesting. A teacher asked a play therapist to come to the school to observe her client, Bobby, a second grader who disrupted the entire class every day with "class clown" behavior. Bobby attended a Catholic school. Although this teacher was quite experienced, she had 36 children in her classroom, and Bobby wanted all of her attention. While observing Bobby in action in the classroom, the play therapist found it hard to imagine how this teacher had been coping with Bobby and his out-of-control behavior for the first 2 months of school. Because Bobby's behavior was all negative-attention-getting, the therapist and teacher developed a classroom time-out behavioral program. In the back of the classroom, the teacher had a corner that was blocked off from the rest of the class with bookshelves and filing cabinets. Teacher and therapist agreed that this would be an appropriate place for a time-out chair. The teacher independently explained to Bobby the new rule: He was not allowed to do anything that would disrupt the class, including calling out, laughing at other children, or calling the teacher's name if he wasn't the first one to be called upon. As part of the plan, the teacher also told Bobby that she would give him one warning about his inappropriate behavior and remind him that if the behavior continued, he would have to go to the time-out chair for 7 minutes (i.e., 1 minute for each year of his age). Because Bobby craved negative attention, the warning and consequence were to be stated in as few words and with as little attention as possible. In order to monitor the effectiveness of the plan, the teacher agreed to record each time she gave Bobby a warning and, if necessary, the time-out consequence. The therapist also cautioned the teacher that Bobby's negative behavior was likely to escalate once he realized that she was regaining control over her classroom.

Things went smoothly the first week, and Bobby spent a fair amount of time in the time-out chair. By the second week, Bobby's behavior started to escalate; he also began singing, "I love going to the time-out chair," when he was given the consequence. The teacher called the therapist one afternoon and frantically proclaimed, "The behavioral program isn't working." She then described Bobby's new antics. A review of the teacher's chart of Bobby's behavior revealed a predictable pattern. The therapist encouraged the teacher to "stay the course" and to continue doing exactly the same thing she had been doing, while ignoring Bobby's singing. By the end of the following week, Bobby's negative-attention-getting behavior was almost extinguished. During that same week, Bobby admitted to his play therapist that although he had told the teacher he liked going to time out, he really didn't. The teacher was relieved to hear Bobby's admission, though neither adult shared this with Bobby. She also expressed gratitude for the therapist's help and support. The therapist congratulated her on her patience with the CCPT process and willingness to work as a team, which served to further Bobby's progress in treatment.

Other School-Related Issues

Parents look to child therapists as experts in all the disturbances of childhood. Because therapists often serve as the "point persons" in managing the overall well-being of children, they should have a working knowledge of all prevalent disorders and other problems that can affect children's behavior, learning, and emotions. For example, an effective CCPT therapist needs to recognize the symptoms of attention-deficit/hyperactivity disorder (ADHD), childhood bipolar disorder, specific learning disabilities, central auditory or visual processing disorders, Asperger syndrome, selective mutism, Tourette syndrome, sensorimotor integration disorder, and physical or sexual abuse. Therapists need not be experts in all of these, but they do need to identify their possible existence and to direct parents to the appropriate referral resources. Upon making such referrals, therapists should keep in touch with these other professionals, to gain information that may affect CCPT and parent consultations. If therapists are not qualified to test for these related childhood problems themselves, it is their obligation to find the resources needed to have children evaluated and treated for them.

In conjunction with parents and teachers, CCPT therapists can also play an important role in developing individualized educational programs (IEPs) for the children with whom they work. Parents are sometimes at a loss as to how to navigate the educational system to obtain special services their child may need. After hearing from parents about school-related issues and working with children in CCPT, therapists often have information that is critical in developing IEPs and planning for educational success. Although therapists usually are not educational law specialists, they can be instrumental in identifying educational advocates or attorneys who can help parents pursue mediation or due process in an effort to obtain an appropriate education for their children, when such measures are needed. Although these issues may appear to be vast endeavors to the novice CCPT therapist, many resources are available to help therapists obtain the knowledge they need to address the needs of children holistically.

Confidentiality and Consent to Treatment

Children under the age of consent (which varies in different states and countries) technically have no rights to confidentiality, as parents can be privy to all their records. This *does not* mean that CCPT therapists must share with parents all the nuances of children's play or what the children reveal during play sessions. Children's privacy can be respected while still keeping parents informed of play themes, the stage of play in which the children are engaged, and the progress being made. Prior to any discussion of children's play sessions with parents, it is worthwhile to help parents understand that children like a certain degree of privacy. Thus, when therapists speak to them about their children, parents need to understand that the discussion should not be revealed to the children and that the children should not be questioned or chastised for what they are doing in play therapy sessions. Also, parents often need to be reminded that children should not be privy to discussions about them either between the parents or with grandparents or other relatives who want to hear the details of the therapy process. Parents need to understand the critical importance of the development of trust in the child–therapist relationship, which can be damaged by comments made to others about a child's therapy within earshot of the child.

Therapists should become familiar with the age of consent in their state, province, or country, and with the implications of this for child treatment. In some cases, children above the age of consent will need to sign a release of information in order for the therapist to discuss their sessions with parents. This becomes an important issue with adolescent clients. All three authors have conducted CCPT and other play interventions with adolescents, sometimes as old as 17 or 18, because the teens found play sessions more comfortable than traditional talk therapy.

In cases where parents are separated or divorced but share legal custody of a child (i.e., the ability to make decisions for the child about health care, education, therapy, etc.), both parents must give written consent for the child to participate in therapy of any kind. This varies by location as well, but therapists have had their licenses to practice threatened by disgruntled parents who did not sign the consent to treatment and later took action against the therapists. If one parent is unwilling to give this consent, the parent desiring therapy for the child can petition the court for permission to have the child receive treatment. This type of petition is rarely turned down, as the courts recognize the importance of getting help for children during difficult periods such as separation or divorce.

Before sending a parent off to file a petition with the court, however, a therapist may find it useful to try to speak to the parent who is refusing treatment, empathically listen to that parent's concerns, and give the rationale for why CCPT is appropriate or is the treatment of choice for these issues. The parent who is refusing treatment may also fear that he or she will not be included, and may need reassurance that the therapist will not give preferential treatment to one parent over the other. Such a conversation frequently results in the parent's agreeing to give consent. There are many reasons why divorced parents are reluctant to consent to treatment, and empathic therapists can usually reassure them once they understand the underlying concerns. Although petitioning the court may be the only recourse in some cases, it sometimes results in a judge's deciding that a new therapist who is acceptable to both parents be engaged—or, in cases of total deadlock between the parents, in the judge's choosing the therapist for the child.

In cases where the parent refusing treatment is suspected of child abuse, therapists may recommend a thorough child abuse evaluation to confirm or rule out the allegation prior to the start of treatment, being careful not to take sides until a final determination is made. In cases where a determination of child abuse is made, the abusing parent generally has his or her legal custody terminated, thereby allowing the parent who has retained legal custody the power to engage the child in whatever treatment the parent deems appropriate. In these types of cases, CCPT therapists must be careful not to confound treatment with evaluation. If they are conducting therapy, then another qualified professional should be performing the child abuse or custody evaluations.

Summary

In summary, it is vital to include parents in the CCPT process. There are many ways to do this, from regular consultations to behavior management to parent skills training to full partnership in FT (see Chapter 8). Parents and teachers have important information to share that helps therapists understand and make better treatment decisions concerning the child. When therapists feel uncomfortable working with parents, the discomfort is likely to be a signal that they would benefit from further training in engagement and collaboration processes with adults. Most parents want to be good parents. They may not know how, and play therapists can play an instrumental role in helping them. Most therapists who genuinely try to be empathic and accepting with parents are pleasantly surprised at how many of them really want to be part of the CCPT process.

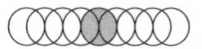

CHAPTER 8

Filial Therapy

Closely related to CCPT is FT, a family therapy method developed by Bernard and Louise Guerney and their colleagues, initially at Rutgers University and later at The Pennsylvania State University (B. G. Guerney, 1964; B. G. Guerney & Guerney, 1961; B. G. Guerney, Stollak, & Guerney, 1970; B. G. Guerney & Stover, 1971). FT offers the best of two worlds: It provides children with all the benefits of CCPT, while involving parents in the process in the fullest possible way. Competence and experience in CCPT are prerequisites for learning FT, and a brief description of FT is included here because it represents the CCPT therapist's next level of professional development.

FT is based on a psychoeducational model (B. G. Guerney, Stollak, & Guerney, 1971), in which parents are first trained in CCPT skills and then use those skills to help their own children overcome emotional and behavioral problems. In essence, parents serve as psychotherapeutic agents, under the supervision of a well-trained FT therapist, to assist their children in overcoming problems. An added benefit is that as parents learn the principles and skills of CCPT, they are assembling a tool-box of skills they can use to relate to their children in productive ways throughout their lifetimes. Furthermore, it is cost-effective for parents.

In the initial stage of FT, therapists teach and supervise parents as they conduct special child-centered play sessions with each of their children (or modified "special times" with adolescents). Half-hour play sessions are held weekly. When parents develop competence and confidence in conducting these under the therapist's direct supervision, they shift to the home environment, where they conduct the play sessions more independently; the FT therapist continues to monitor the home play sessions via parents' reports or videos. The final stage of FT involves helping the parents generalize their use of the CCPT skills to daily life. Initially therapists ask parents to confine their use of the CCPT skills to the parent–child play sessions until they have mastered them sufficiently to generalize them, but it is quite common for parents to "admit" that they have tried the skills in the home environment outside the play sessions, in advance of the final generalization process. This suggests the motivational benefits of working collaboratively with parents, but perhaps even more important are parents' reports that they found the skills so useful that they could not wait to apply them in their day-to-day parenting. It is gratifying for therapists when parents recognize the value of the child-centered skills in this way!

The FT process is described in much greater detail elsewhere (L. F. Guerney, 1976, 1983; VanFleet, 2005, 2006b, 2008a; VanFleet & Guerney, 2003; Sywulak, 2003; VanFleet & Sniscak, 2003a, 2003b). Adaptations of the Guerneys' original and complete family therapy model are also available (Landreth & Bratton, 2006; Caplin & Pernet, in press; VanFleet & Sniscak, in press; Wright & Walker, 2003). Research has clearly demonstrated the effectiveness of FT in facilitating long-term, whole-family change (Bratton et al., 2005; VanFleet, Ryan, & Smith, 2005).

The Value of FT to Children

Play therapists who are practitioners of CCPT recognize its value and power. All therapists who are committed to this nondirective model have many stories to tell of their successes and the wonderful ways in which children find their own paths to healthy functioning, good self-esteem, and self-responsibility. However, as much as we three authors love conducting CCPT, we all have found that the use of FT usually outweighs the benefits of doing CCPT individually with children. Although this book is devoted to the effective practice of CCPT, it is closely linked with the practice of FT. There are several reasons for the value of FT in child therapy.

Child therapists, even those who see children frequently for years, can never surpass or even duplicate the relationships children have with their parents—nor should that be an objective. The natural bond between a parent and child affords the parent a level of trust and connection with the child that cannot be undone. Even when a parent violates the child's trust, such as in cases of physical or sexual abuse, that child yearns for the parent's love and attention. This is not intended to imply that play therapists' relationships with the children with whom they work are insignificant. Experienced CCPT therapists typically create strong relationships and trust that cannot be easily broken. Even so, therapists' work with children always comes to an end. Those children return to parents (or other family members or guardians) who, in the best circumstances, will continue using the parenting and behavior skills they have learned as part of their involvement in the children's therapy. These parents don't have the full advantage of learning CCPT skills in an intensive and supervised setting, however, as they would in FT. FT enables parents to practice and *master* skills that will become part of who they are as parents, but this is not true when therapists' time is devoted primarily to individual CCPT sessions with the children. When children are seen in individual therapy, it is more likely that they will return to therapy in later years if new problems arise for which their parents feel unprepared. Furthermore, children benefit from the increased security and attunement within the enhanced parent–child attachment that FT makes possible. Years of research have shown that children make significant and long-lasting changes when their parents engage in the process of FT with them (B. G. Guerney & Stover, 1971; Sywulak, 1978; Sensue, 1981; Bratton et al., 2005; VanFleet et al., 2005).

The Value of FT to Parents

FT is designed to teach parents lifelong parenting skills, which they practice and master by learning CCPT. The FT process, at its best, gives the therapist a much clearer window into the world of parents and their children. The nature of the supervised parent–child play sessions reveals family dynamics to the therapist. Family intervention then becomes an active process, in which the therapist provides direct feedback to parents about their skill acquisition and addresses the parent–child issues and/or psychodynamics that underlie the problems the family is experiencing. Such was the case with a single father and his two boys, ages 8 and 11, who participated in FT.

The father, John, had left the marriage after much marital discord and many failed attempts in marital therapy. Close to the time of separation, his wife lost a well-paying job and had serious bouts of depression. The boys, Mark and Daniel, were furious at their father for leaving, especially since their mother was struggling with so many problems of her own. The separation and pending divorce, paired with the mother's dramatic loss of income, meant that the family home had to be sold; neither parent could afford to keep the house as a single parent. The boys' world had been turned upside down, and they simply could not understand how their father could leave, triggering this dramatic change in their lives. The boys were further confused about the separation, because they had never seen their parents fighting. The parents somehow had managed to shield the children from their serious problems by reserving their disputes for their sessions with a string of marriage therapists. FT seemed important to help the father rebuild his relationship with Mark and Daniel while helping them work through their strong and confused feelings.

Once John began in-office parent–child play sessions, it readily became apparent how emotionally shut down he had become. As the boys acted out their intense anger in the playroom, the father remained calm and aloof. By questioning the boys about neutral topics during the play session, the father tried to move the boys away from their angry feelings. Needless to say, the father's failure to empathically understand his children was interfering in their ability to process their anger. After a couple of sessions of providing skills feedback to this father about his difficulty in accepting and reflecting the boys' anger, the FT therapist decided to intervene empathically with him in the post-play-session discussion period. She acknowledged to John how anxious he was in the playroom when it came to understanding and accepting the boys' anger. Her empathy and acceptance of his feelings opened many doors for this father, as he discussed how both he and his wife had not been able to express their own anger toward each other appropriately and had spent most of their time pretending nothing was wrong between them. John also revealed that he had been raised by a rageful alcoholic father, and John had vowed that he would never be like him. In other words, John had learned to fear anger and learned to manage his fear by avoiding expressions of anger through denial and distraction. The breakthrough came when the father realized how his unwillingness to accept his own sons' anger was keeping them stuck in an angry place and undermining the relationship he so desperately wanted to have with them.

While conducting child-centered play sessions with their children, parents are amazed at how much they learn about their children—and, perhaps more importantly, about themselves. The work children do in the nondirective play sessions with their own parents opens doors for the parents to experience who they are as people and as parents at the deepest levels. At some very basic level, children simply know how to give parents the experience they need to understand family dynamics, parental inadequacies, the nature of the parent–child relationship, and what needs to change in the family to make it truly functional. The problem is that until parents learn how to conduct FT play sessions, they often are not "tuned in" at a deep level and simply miss the messages children are trying to convey. FT affords these parents the skills and the opportunity to do just that. That learning can be quite powerful, as evidenced in a case involving an 8-year-old boy, Timothy, who entered the world of play with his parents through FT in the 1970s.

Timothy was a perfectionistic child who had poor self-esteem and a low threshold for frustration. He was doing poorly in school, had no friends, and often told his parents he was so unhappy that he wished he were dead. The parents were lovely people and eager to learn the skills of CCPT to help their son. They arrived promptly for each group FT session—the father dressed in expensive slacks and a white dress shirt, and the mother dressed in the most fashionable pant suits. Their fingernails were manicured, and every hair of their stylish coiffures was in place. They stood out in stark contrast to the other parents in the group, who were more typical '70s parents—casually dressed in blue jeans and T-shirts or sweatshirts, depending on the weather. Timothy was a spiffy kid, too; he looked like a younger version of his parents. During demonstration play sessions conducted by the therapist, Timothy was awkward and uncomfortable with the freedom of the "special room." He would often wait for direction from the therapist, who reminded him that he was free to do almost anything he wanted in the special room. Mostly, he explored the playroom very cautiously during the demonstration sessions.

What a surprise the group received when Timothy had his first play session with his mother! Upon entering the playroom, Timothy asked his mother, dressed in her stylish pant suit, to get down on her hands and knees. He then proceeded to tie the jump rope loosely around his mother's neck, and told her to follow him around the room and moo like a cow as he led her by the rope he held. Timothy's mother was an ace! She followed his directions to the letter and reflected his feelings of delight at being in charge in the special room. Whenever Timothy told her to keep mooing, she would moo for a while longer and then empathically listen to his feelings again. Two FT therapists, Timothy's father, and four other parents from the group watched this play unfold. Everyone behind the one-way mirror giggled at the scene and commented how well the mother was handling Timothy's symbolic play.

After the play session, the mother and others returned to the meeting room to discuss Timothy's play session. The FT therapists and the other parents told her what a wonderful job she had done under circumstances that would ordinarily embarrass a parent. Timothy's mother was appreciative of the comments, but started to cry. She explained that she now understood how much pressure she had put on Timothy and her family to be picture-perfect, and how she was probably transmitting her own insecurities and feelings of not being "good enough" to them. The FT therapists listened attentively and empathically as this mother, through her reflections on what she had just learned from her son, began to open doors for herself and her family that could lead to positive change. It was an emotional session for everyone, but valuable lessons were learned about what children can teach adults through the CCPT skills of attention, attunement, and acceptance.

The learning that occurred during this session was immediately evident when the group met the following week. At the next session, Timothy's parents arrived a little early, dressed in blue jeans and casual shirts. They were eager to share how different Timothy's mood had been over the past week, and how they felt as if they could finally relax and enjoy each other without having to pretend to be the perfect family. What a lesson everyone learned from a child who asked his mother, in the context of nondirective parent–child play, to be a cow and moo!

Conducting FT

When FT was first conceived by the Guerneys in the early 1960s, it was conducted in a group format, usually consisting of six parents. This group format offers significant advantages. It provides a support system for parents, as they quickly learn that they are not alone in the struggles with their children. Also, the parents benefit from watching other parents learn the CCPT skills and from being able to participate, as modeled by the FT therapists, in observing and reinforcing the accomplishments of the other parents. This phenomenon is best explained by what has been called the "helper therapy principle," which was first described by Frank Reissman (1965). According to this theory, in the process of helping other group members, the group members who are helping gain an increased sense of self-efficacy and mastery. Results of Reissman's work revealed that taking both helper and helpee roles in a group with mutual concerns was correlated with improved psychological well-being and perceived benefits of the group.

Unfortunately, the group format is not often feasible in many clinic or private practice settings, simply because of the logistics of getting several parents together in one room on any given night for a period of 18–24 weeks. Therefore, a 10-session model (90-minute sessions) with individual families was developed for use in settings not conducive to the original group format (Ginsberg, 1997; Sywulak, 2003). Others have utilized shorter sessions (1 hour) over longer periods in a 15- to 20-session model (VanFleet, 2005, 2006b). In addition, FT has been used as a home-based intervention, in which a therapist travels with a kit of toys and conducts FT in the home from the start (VanFleet, 2005). Shorter-term group models have also been developed for a variety of applications (Caplin & Pernet, in press; Landreth & Bratton, 2006; VanFleet & Sniscak, in press; Wright & Walker, 2003).

Although conducting FT in an individual format means that the model loses some of the richness of the group experience, the individual family approach affords the therapist and the family the opportunity to address some family and even marital issues at deeper levels than can be accomplished in a group, and over a shorter period of time. The efficacy of FT has been demonstrated in many settings, such as private practices, clinics, schools, day care settings, prisons, and hospitals. These variations in setting and differing formats serve to highlight how robust the FT approach actually is.

The Importance of Training in FT

As noted at the beginning of this chapter, good training and supervised experience in CCPT are prerequisites for learning to conduct FT. Although FT employs the skills of CCPT, it is distinctly different in that it is based on an educational model. This means that the FT therapist must understand how to balance the didactic or teaching components of the model with the dynamic aspects, which are addressed largely from a client-centered stance. In FT, parents are treated with respect and appreciation, and are viewed as "experts" on their children. Understanding and accepting the parents' feelings with genuine regard for them as people and parents are at the core of building a therapeutic relationship, as well as means to help parents identify and resolve intra- and interpersonal issues that may be interfering with their learning. The didactic skills include brief lecturing, demonstrations, modeling, structuring, exercises, role playing, shaping, social reinforcement, and skill generalization.

Like CCPT, FT may appear to be a rather straightforward approach, but both CCPT and FT have nuances in their methods that can be learned only through good training and supervision. As we know from our experiences as supervisors and instructors, simply reading a book or watching a video does not constitute sufficient training for the effective use of these methods.

Where to Get Training in FT

We have all offered training in FT to thousands of therapists in the United States and abroad. Sometimes universities, institutes, or mental health agencies establish a training venue by forming a group of interested participants and importing the FT instructors. Some therapists have initially learned CCPT with their own children in a place of treatment, and then have sought FT training through a qualified trainer.

Our contact information is listed in Chapter 14 for ease of accessing our client services, supervision, and training programs. All of us use the Guerney-based CCPT and FT methods that we learned directly from the Guerneys and have written about in this volume. In addition, the National Institute of Relationship Enhancement (NIRE; *www.nire. org*) was established by the Guerneys to provide services to professionals. The NIRE website offers an extensive list of publications and videos. Many other centers and universities now offer training courses in FT, and readers may contact us about these or review the resources listed below. Professionals may now pursue credentials such as -Certified Filial Therapist and Certified Filial Therapy Instructor (*www.play-therapy. com*).

Other Sources of Information about FT

Key resources about the original Guerney-based approach to FT are listed below. Details are provided in the References list at the end of this book.

- Books

  - *Filial Therapy: Strengthening Parent–Child Relationships through Play* (2nd ed.) (VanFleet, 2005)
  - *Casebook of Filial Therapy* (VanFleet & Guerney, 2003)
  - *Relationship Enhancement Family Therapy* (Ginsberg, 1997)

- DVDs

  - *Introduction to Filial Therapy* (VanFleet, 2006b)
  - *Filial Play Therapy* (VanFleet, 2008a)

PART IV

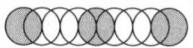

PRACTICAL APPLICATIONS AND ISSUES

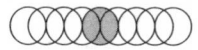

CHAPTER 9

Child-Centered Play Therapy
with Different Presenting Problems

CCPT is a process-oriented approach to intervention. As such, it has considerable usefulness for many different types of presenting problems. Often very little change to the basic approach is needed. As long as clinicians adhere to Axline's eight principles (see Chapter 3) and follow the skill guidelines (see Chapter 5), the approach can be applied with very little adjustment. Most of the time, adaptations are related more to a particular physical environment or setting than to the methodology of CCPT. As long as therapists have access to a space they can use as a playroom and to a variety of toys, they can structure, empathically listen, engage in child-centered imaginary play when invited, and set limits with children.

It seems useful for readers to take a closer look at what happens in CCPT and FT. This can provide a greater understanding of the scope and depth that the CCPT approach offers, while demonstrating how the methods are used with different child and family problems. There are as many variations in children's play during CCPT and FT as there are children. The case vignettes in this chapter are representative of that variety. They are organized under headings reflecting the primary reasons for referral, although many of the children depicted had multiple difficulties.

It is important to note that when children are very distressed and/ or have complicated emotional, social, and behavioral issues, as often happens in cases of abuse and neglect, they often need a comprehensive, multimodal treatment program. One type of intervention is rarely enough. In these cases, CCPT or FT can form the core of their treatment, but many other interventions are often employed as well. To stay within the scope of this volume, we have provided information only about the CCPT and FT portions of treatment.

In order to protect the clients' privacy, identifying information in the case vignettes has been changed (as it has in all case material used in this book). Most of the case examples are composites of several different families. The clinical problems, play session behaviors and themes, family dynamics, and interventions realistically illustrate CCPT and FT principles, however.

Anxiety

Anxiety in children occurs for many reasons, and it can interfere with daily life at times. Sometimes there is considerable anxiety in the family system, but sometimes the anxiety stems from peer relations, difficulties or pressures related to school, or frightening events in children's lives. Many parents report that their efforts to console or distract their children through words and reasoning have no effect. CCPT is often useful for anxiety, as it allows children to express their feelings and gain mastery over their fears in a personally meaningful way. Two examples follow.

Alison, age 8, was referred for play therapy because of her anxiety after her grandfather died. She had not attended the funeral, but thereafter she told her parents about nightmares involving caskets, dead people, burials, and devils. During her first CCPT session, she noticed some clear masks that had just a small amount of color on the lips and over the eye holes. She looked away quickly, said, "I don't like those," and asked the therapist to place them on a high shelf. The therapist did as asked. Alison was then able to play—often with the kitchen set, preparing meals and washing the toy dishes. Each of her first five play sessions started the same way, with her request for the therapist to place the masks high and out of sight. As she entered the playroom on her sixth visit, she picked up one of the masks, handed it to the therapist, and motioned for the therapist to put it on. The therapist did so, and Alison laughed. She then put the other mask on herself, looked in the mirror, and laughed again. From that point onward, she seemed unconcerned about the masks. They apparently had lost their frightening quality when she was able to control them via the therapist. Alison participated in 12 CCPT sessions, coupled with some grief activities at home. The home activities involved putting together a memory book of her grandfather, including a photo from the actual funeral and several drawings Alison made. Her anxiety and nightmares disappeared.

Tony, 5 years old, was brought to play therapy after he was in a car accident with his mother. He was injured only slightly, but his mother sustained a potentially serious neck injury, and she was placed in an ambulance and taken to the hospital. A policewoman on the scene stayed with Tony until his father arrived. His mother was hospitalized overnight and released; she attended physical therapy and made a quick recovery. Tony seemed fine, except that the parents noted he was quieter than he had been before the accident.

A month after the accident, the family was driving through town and saw an ambulance in the oncoming traffic. There was a short blast of the siren, and the lights were flashing. Tony immediately began screaming and thrashing in the back seat. His parents' efforts to calm him down had no effect, and his highly distressed behavior continued for nearly an hour. The next day, when the family was watching a television program, the emergency vehicles that came onscreen triggered another intense reaction. Tony then showed reactivity to every exposure he had to emergency vehicles—in real life, on television, and even in news magazine photographs. After trying unsuccessfully to handle this for several months, his parents sought help. Although FT would have been appropriate for this family, the mother still had some mobility problems, and the father's job took him out of town frequently. The therapist and parents jointly decided that they would start with CCPT and postpone FT for a few months.

In the first CCPT session, Tony barely spoke to the therapist. He explored the playroom and touched or played with several different toys. He did not stay with any item for long. The therapist reflected his exploration: "You're checking out those army guys. . . . You just found the guns and are trying to see how they work. . . . Pow! Hitting that bag. . . . You think that mask is funny. . . . Oooo, you don't like that one at all. . . . Whamo! You bopped that bag again. You like the way that feels. . . . Feeling that sand, letting it run through your fingers. . . . "

In his second play session, Tony explored some more and then settled by the sandtray. He took some miniature medical characters and created an operating room scene in the sand. He also placed a female figure in a hospital bed. Once again, the therapist reflected what he was doing and any feelings he was expressing: "Looks like you're setting up something. . . . That doctor just put on his mask. Oh, there are two people working on the lady. They are trying lots of different things on her. They seem worried about how she is doing." At this last comment, Tony looked at the therapist and nodded his head. From that point onward, he narrated his own play: "This is the thing that goes over the face to make people sleep. . . . The lady is sleeping, and they are fixing her." Tony spent nearly the entire session creating this medical scene, which seemed related to his fears about what had happened to his mother after the accident.

In his third play session, Tony selected a large floppy doll and put the stethoscope around his neck. He announced that he was the doctor and that the therapist was the nurse. He pointed to the doll and said he had to check out his patient. Following his instructions, the therapist held the doll while Tony checked its heart and blood pressure, using the toy medical kit. Next Tony said, "Now I have to check the flexes. Nurse, hand me the hammer." The therapist, playing the nurse role, handed him an instrument and said, "Here's your hammer, Doctor." Tony then hit the knee of the doll as if checking reflexes. He took the floppy leg and kicked it high into the air. He continued to check both knees of his "patient" many times. The therapist, still in the nurse role, said, "Wow, Doctor, you sure have to check out those flexes! You're making sure that patient is all right." For the rest of the session, Tony had a wrestling match with the bop bag.

Tony returned to the doctor play in his fourth CCPT session, again checking the knee reflexes, the heart, and blood pressure. This time he pretended to give injections in many places on the doll. At the 5-minute warning, he took out the ambulance, pressed the button that turned on the lights, and drove it around the room. He placed the oversized doll on top of it and drove it some more.

The therapist believed that the medical play was directly related to Tony's fears surrounding the accident, especially the injury and separation from his mother. He increasingly took charge of the play, suggesting gradual mastery of his fears. At the same time, his parents reported that he was becoming less reactive to emergency vehicles and had asked to see some of the news magazine pictures again. He looked at them carefully and did not have a "meltdown" as he had before.

In subsequent play sessions, Tony continued his doctor and ambulance play. By his ninth play session, he asked the therapist to play the role of an ambulance person along with him. Following his lead, the therapist rushed to the side of the floppy doll, who had fallen down and needed assistance. After this session, Tony no longer engaged in medical play; instead, he played with the bop bag, the kitchen set, and the dinosaurs. His parents reported no further incidents of emergency-reactive behaviors. It seemed that Tony had mastered his anxieties by taking charge in his play, and that he now felt more in control of himself.

Divorce

Divorce usually is confusing for children. They feel attachments to both parents, and the loss of daily contact (or sometimes of any contact at all) with one can shake their sense of security. Many feelings can surface, and when parents are caught up in their own emotional reactions, they sometimes fail to see their children's distress. CCPT can offer children of divorce an opportunity to express their feelings, master their fears, and adjust to the changed living arrangements and the sometimes volatile relationships of their parents.

Diane's mother and father were divorced. She and her younger brother lived with their mother, and at first had regular visits with their father. The father had a history of substance abuse and domestic violence. The police had been called to their home many times in the past, and Diane and her brother had witnessed these episodes. On one of the children's visits, their father got high and passed out. Diane, who was 7 years old at the time, had to call emergency services. When the police arrived, their father was belligerent and aggressive. After this, the court suspended the father's visits and awarded full custody to the mother. The father then harassed the family, usually when under the influence of drugs or alcohol, and he ranted and raved at the children over the phone. He also threatened to come and take the children away from their mother. Diane felt unsafe much of the time, but she also expressed worries that she had been responsible for the family difficulties and she wished that her parents would reunite. She was frequently anxious, and continually checked to be sure that the doors and windows were locked.

She refused to talk with her father by phone, but afterward she felt guilty about "hurting his feelings."

Diane's mother was extremely stressed, especially during the prolonged custody battle that ensued. She faced financial problems and relied on extended family members for help with the children. Indeed, she was so stressed and depressed that FT was not indicated at the time. The therapist therefore used CCPT to work with Diane. In the first session, Diane decided to work on an art project. She appeared cautious, using the time to determine whether the therapist and the playroom provided a safe environment wherein she could do her work. She did not talk about any issues related to her family. During the second CCPT session, Diane spent considerable time moving sand back and forth in the sandtray, saying that she was bored and could not find anything to do. The therapist stayed reflective, empathic, and attentive to her. At the 5-minute warning signaling the end of the play session, Diane selected some animal figures for the sandtray. She placed angry- and scary-looking animals in one area, and several family units of woodland and domestic animals in a separate area across from the angry animals. The session then ended.

In her third CCPT session 2 weeks later, Diane went directly to the sandtray. She told the therapist that she wanted to keep working on the sandtray she had started in the second session. She spent much of the session finding the figures she wanted, discarding some because they did not fit the plan she had in mind. She eventually chose a lion, a tiger, a gorilla, and many snakes. She said, "I hate snakes. They scare me." She picked up a giraffe and asked the therapist, "Are they nice?" The therapist reflected the question: "You're trying to tell if they're nice." Diane then put the giraffe aside, saying, "No . . . they are too kind and gentle." She wanted only scary, aggressive, and mean animals on one side.

She constructed a large barrier out of sand, and on the other side of this hill she made a home for the families of the other animals: bunnies, squirrels, deer, owls, and raccoons. She identified the members of each family as mother, father, and children. She also carefully placed furniture around the animal families. She explained that they needed nice places to sleep and watch television. She placed the adult animals in beds, the child animals in another place, and the baby animals in cribs. The therapist reflected, "You're making a nice and comfortable home for the animals." Diane responded, "Yes, but they have no idea what will happen tomorrow." This comment seemed to reveal her anxiety about the lack of control she felt on a daily basis. It seemed that she was trying to create a more comfortable and protected environment for the animal families, much as she probably needed herself. Diane then stated that the animals could climb to the top of the hill and see what was coming. She seemed to be giving them a greater sense of control over the unknown threats posed by the mean animals on the other side. She indicated that the family animals did not like being scared.

Next Diane giggled as she selected some miniature boxes wrapped as shiny gifts, with many colored bows on top. She told the therapist that they were actually bombs. The therapist responded, using the empathic listening skill, "Oh, secret weapons—they won't know they are bombs." Diane laughed again and said, "They won't know what hit them."

After everything was set up to her satisfaction and the therapist had given the 5-minute warning, the aggressive characters started to move closer to the top of the hill. The family members on the other side were in their beds and watching television when the attack began. Diane quickly took all the child figures and placed them in the crib, saying, "They will be safe there." Then all of the adult family animals threw the gift boxes over the hill at the attackers. One by one, the aggressors died. Diane turned all of the attackers upside down in the sand until they were all dead. She smiled and laughed as she did this. The therapist reflected: "They did not know what they were going to get. These little animals tricked them. Even though they were little, they were strong and powerful and found a way to stay safe and protect themselves." When all the aggressors had been hit by the presents/bombs, Diane announced, "I'm done." She seemed visibly more relaxed and left the playroom.

It is interesting that Diane seemed to come to the playroom with a plan, prepared to work. She spent most of the session deciding how to implement her plan. The conquering of the attackers was actually a very brief moment in the session. It appeared that the planning and sense of mastery she gained from developing the story helped relieve much of her anxiety. She was able symbolically to gain a sense of power and control over the victimization and sense of helplessness that these animals felt, much as she had felt within her family.

Diane's mother reported that she seemed much less anxious at home after this session, further suggesting that she had attained some mastery over the frightening feelings she had experienced. She continued to use the CCPT sessions to work through some additional concerns, but she did the bulk of her needed work in these first three sessions. She required only 10 sessions of CCPT after the intake process.

Attention-Deficit/Hyperactivity Disorder

It is quite common for children with ADHD to experience problems at school and home. In addition to the difficulties posed by the symptoms of ADHD, they often struggle with relationships, feelings of frustration, and poor self-concept. CCPT helps these children with their feelings and self-concepts, and FT can be very useful for smoothing out parent–child and family relationships. Other, more directive play therapy interventions can be useful in addressing specific symptoms or goal areas (see Kaduson, 2006).

Brent was 9 years old when his father brought him for therapy. He was having increasing periods of oppositionality, tantrums, and physical fights with his younger brother. When he went through periods of misbehavior, he took things that did not belong to him and made up stories when questioned about it. Brent and his brother were both adopted, and his brother had serious visual impairment and some neurological problems. Brent was tall, physically agile, and full of energy. Because of this, many people expected more of him than was realistic for his chronological age. It seemed that he frequently fell short of others' expectations. Complicating this, his younger brother's misbehaviors were often forgiven because "he couldn't help it," but Brent was presumed to know better.

Brent loved CCPT. His play frequently included one particular activity: He would set the playroom up as a soccer field and ask the therapist to serve as the opposing team. He enjoyed making up the rules and changing them to meet his needs. If it appeared that he was winning too much, he would allow the therapist to score a couple of times. Winning was important for him, and in the end, he always won the matches. He was very competitive and enjoyed outsmarting the therapist. He came up with creative ways to "distract" the therapist while he ran down the "field" and scored, and he seemed pleased with himself when he succeeded. He always played with great energy and enthusiasm.

Brent's treatment plan also included other types of play therapy, but the CCPT seemed very useful for him. His play themes included self-esteem, mastery, power and control, capable identity, limit testing, competition, aggression, winning, relationship, and problem solving. This type of play allowed him to be physically active and engaged. He had few opportunities for this at home, and most real-world play carried with it many adult expectations for conformity and "playing by the rules." His larger size often meant that he played games and sports with older children, among whom he had little chance of success because of his age, impulsivity, and distractibility. Being permitted to change the rules in CCPT was novel; it allowed him to feel competent, capable, and proud of himself. He used the sessions to explore and accept himself in a way that was not possible in the often critical family environment. He always left the playroom a happy child, and his behavior improved after each session. His father reported less aggression and oppositionality at home following his CCPT sessions. The directive play therapy interventions increased his focus and reduced his impulsivity somewhat. The therapist wanted to involve the family in FT, but plans for the family to move into a new home prevented this from occurring.

Developmental Disability

Lucy was 15 when she was referred for play therapy. She had a developmental disability and lived in a foster home. She had been removed from her mother because of neglect, and she also had a history of sexual and physical abuse. She attended a special education class in the high school. She expressed the desire to be like other children her age; she often talked about music, hair styling, and makeup.

A major concern for Lucy's foster mother was that Lucy carried a baby doll to school. When forbidden to do so, she hid it in her backpack. It seemed that she needed this doll to get through her day. The foster mother was concerned about the age-appropriateness of this and feared that Lucy would be teased by the other students.

Lucy used the CCPT sessions to work through much of her historical abuse. One day, after learning that her biological mother's parental rights had been terminated, Lucy picked up a baby bottle and pretended to put it in her mouth. She looked warily at the therapist, appearing somewhat embarrassed. The therapist reflected her uncertainty: "You're wondering if it's okay for you to use the bottle." (This therapist used separate nipples for each child to permit drinking from the bottle, as we have described in Chapter 5.) Lucy smiled and put it in her mouth. The therapist said, "Sometimes it feels good to be a baby." Lucy lay down on the floor and curled into a fetal position. The therapist sat on a small chair a few feet away. Lucy continued to suck on the bottle in this position. She asked the therapist to sing. The therapist sang a soothing lullaby, as one might do with an infant. Lucy remained in this position for the 10 remaining minutes of the session, sometimes making baby noises. The therapist continued softly singing or humming except when giving the 5- and 1-minute time warnings. When the session was over, Lucy calmly arose and left the playroom. She engaged in the same type of regressive play for the next two sessions; after this, she stopped carrying her baby doll to school. It seemed as if Lucy had been reparenting herself by creating the nurturance she had never received from a primary caregiver.

Attachment Problems

Attachment problems can be extremely challenging for families. They are usually entwined with abuse or other trauma, and children's behaviors can be frightening and extreme. The usual parenting methods do not seem to work well, if at all. By the time parents come for therapy, they can be exhausted. CCPT is useful in helping children learn to express and manage their feelings and to develop better self-regulation. FT is particularly useful in helping the entire family build healthy attachment at the same time that the trauma issues are addressed (VanFleet, 2006c; VanFleet & Sniscak, 2003a, in press).

Brittany was brought to therapy by her mother when she was 12. She was an African American adopted into a European American family; there were two other adopted children in the family. Brittany had lived with the family as a foster child since she was 5 years old, and the parents had adopted her when she was 9 years old. She had a long history of misbehavior. Felicia, the mother, reported that Brittany was oppositional, stole and hoarded food, lied, fought with her siblings, and took things that did not belong to her. She also did not get along with peers at school. Brittany was a capable student, but had been placed in an emotional support classroom. She had prior diagnoses of ADHD and reactive attachment disorder. Her history prior to being placed in foster care was unclear: Nothing was known about her parents, but, despite the lack of historical information, abuse was suspected.

Felicia and her husband were very frustrated with Brittany's behaviors, which upset the entire family. Felicia reported that she was unable to leave Brittany alone for even a few minutes, because she could not be trusted. Brittany's parents were so frustrated with the accumulated stress that they were considering placing her in a residential treatment center, and they had told her this. They came to therapy as a last resort.

Brittany was happy to come to therapy. She told the therapist that her parents did not listen to her. She explained that she was different from others in her family and that she was treated unfairly. She said that sometimes she felt like a prisoner there. She was frequently made to stay in her room alone, and she disliked having to be with one of her parents constantly, with no freedom to play or explore on her own. Brittany told the therapist that she wanted to please her parents and to have good relationships, and it upset her that her mother was often angry with her.

Felicia bore most of the child-rearing responsibilities herself. She was worn out and had little patience left for Brittany's challenges. She believed that Brittany was sabotaging her efforts to be a good parent on a daily basis.

After the initial intake meeting with the parents, the therapist observed Brittany in the playroom with both of her parents. Of significance during this observation session was one point when Brittany dressed in a blonde wig. She posed for her parents and told them that she wished she were light-skinned like the rest of the family. The therapist offered FT to the parents, and they were trained in three sessions.

In Brittany's first play session with Felicia, Brittany dressed in a fancy gown and high-heeled shoes. She dressed Felicia in a purple boa and gave her a purse and play money. Felicia readily entered into the imaginary play. Brittany said that they were going to buy babies. They went to the store, where Brittany selected and named three babies. After a while, she quizzed Felicia to see whether she remembered the unique names, and then rewarded her with money and praise if she did. It seemed as if she were testing to see if Felicia really knew who her children were. Together they changed the babies' diapers, fed them, and then placed them in a small crib to sleep.

Next Brittany invited Felicia to a special buffet. Brittany laid out a big feast, using all the plastic food. She asked Felicia to eat whatever she wished, and Brittany did not eat until she was certain that Felicia was satisfied. She made small talk with her mother (in character) and offered her more play money for gas so she would not have to worry about that. Felicia engaged admirably in the imaginary play of this first session. She stayed within role without leading the play, and she used empathic listening appropriately, identifying some of Brittany's character's feelings.

The themes of this first session seemed to be strongly related to the mother–child relationship and adoption; the general caretaking and nurturing of infants; and the importance of remembering and honoring the uniqueness of each child. Brittany felt rejected and out of place in her family, and this session allowed her to enact the type of attention adopted babies needed. The food play echoed some disagreements at home about eating. In her roles, Brittany was loving, kind, and generous—behaviors that Felicia never noticed at home. Felicia was impressed with Brittany's behaviors during this first session, and she was surprised at how much Brittany enjoyed playing with her.

The second session was quite different. Once again dressed in the gown and heels, Brittany gave her mother a series of weapons and took some for herself. She said, "There ain't room for the two of us," and a mock battle ensued. There was lots of laughter as they hid behind barriers, crossed swords, and threw "bombs" (balls) at each other. When Felicia began to retreat, Brittany said, "Get back here!" The battle ended with mother and child laughing heartily. Felicia once again expressed amazement that Brittany wanted to engage with her in the play sessions. The therapist and Felicia discussed possible themes for the session as including aggression and control (reflecting the real-life battles at home), but also relationship building and Brittany's wish to be part of Felicia's life. Felicia said that this was the first day she had felt hope for Brittany in a very long time.

The third parent–child play session was different from the first two. Brittany asked Felicia to sit in a chair in front of the puppet theater, telling her that she was the "audience." Brittany hid behind the theater and dressed in a fancy silver jacket, a black mask covering her eyes, and a long blonde wig. She emerged from behind the theater with a microphone, singing as if she were a performer. The theme of the song was "We belong together." Initially she sang tentatively, but as her confidence grew, she began belting out the song with passion. Her selection of this song seemed no accident. It appeared that Brittany was trying to be the person she thought her mother wanted, while pleading with her to work things out.

Brittany decided to sing another song and disappeared behind the theater to change her outfit. She reemerged from the dressing area without the mask or wig. She sang again, this time about the inability to be perfect. The song was about someone who tried to please but always fell short—about never being good enough. Felicia played the "audience" as instructed and listened to what Brittany was telling her. In her discussion with the therapist afterward, Felicia said that she wished they had known about FT when Brittany was younger.

These three sessions made a marked difference in the relationship between Felicia and Brittany. Brittany's difficult behaviors were continuing at home, but Felicia began to see them in a different light. Her understanding of the impact of trauma coupled with attachment issues grew, and she began to see the potential of this type of play with her most challenging child. They had much work ahead of them, but the relationship had begun to grow, and Felicia's hope motivated her to continue.

Posttraumatic Stress Disorder

Children experiencing posttraumatic stress disorder (PTSD) have many feelings to work out. They must come to terms with the traumatic situation, and more specifically with the feelings of fear, terror, helplessness, and hopelessness that are the hallmarks of trauma. It is common for children to play out trauma-related themes and feelings early in CCPT. When they feel sufficiently safe and accepted, they typically move into mastery play, in which they overcome these feelings by taking charge of situations. Mastery play often parallels improvements in real-life functioning. CCPT offers children the control they need to overcome the helplessness they have experienced, and the nondirective nature of the therapy permits them to do this in their own ways and at their own pace. This ensures that they take an active role in their own healing— an important feature of recovery from trauma. The play keeps it safe, and the self-directedness builds children's coping and confidence (Van-Fleet & Sniscak, 2003b).

Kirk began therapy when he was 9 years old, after he reported being molested by another child in his foster home. His biological mother was mentally ill, and he had lived with her in a car and a shelter until he was removed from her custody because of domestic violence involving one of his mother's boyfriends, in which his mother and he were injured.

Kirk had many symptoms of PTSD, including fear, hypervigilance, night terrors, crying, lying, stealing, and explosive anger. Most of the time he appeared sad and depressed. He could not get along with his foster siblings, even after the boy who molested him was placed elsewhere. Kirk also missed his mother and worried about her, as he had tried to protect her and keep her safe when she could not care for herself.

Kirk did not want to talk about himself or his experiences. He said very little to the therapist, even when they entered the playroom. He played with miniature toys on the floor, using little space; he spent most of the first session crashing the cars into each other.

After several weeks of CCPT, Kirk's play became more expansive. He continued to play on the floor, but used more space and a greater variety of toys. His play was intricate: He designed entire towns that contained humans and pets. As people in the miniature towns went about their business, these play sequences always contained some element of threat or danger. Children were injured as their buses crashed en route to school. Kirk dispatched emergency and rescue teams, but these helpers usually met with disasters of their own. They never seemed able to protect or help the child victims. There were mayhem and chaos all over town. Homes burned, and fire trucks could not come quickly enough. Bad guys robbed banks, and the police cars crashed while the robbers escaped. Schools were bombed. Hurricanes and tornadoes struck the town, leaving people lost under the debris. Kirk said little to the therapist, although he narrated some of the most dire circumstances and occasionally asked the therapist to assist with some of these play scenes. This play continued for many sessions.

It appeared that the world was a bleak and dangerous place for Kirk. The characters were powerless to save themselves, as were the helpers. The play themes highlighted a sense of helplessness and hopelessness. Bad things could happen at any time, and although there were helpers, they could not help. The scenes Kirk created were filled with fear, victimization, and vulnerability. There was an overriding sense of chaos and disorganization. It should be noted that Kirk was very engaged with the play, often making siren noises, screeching and crashing sounds, and dramatic use of the toys.

During these early sessions, despite the disastrous themes, Kirk's behavior in the world seemed to stabilize. His foster mother reported that his behavior with the other children was improving, and that he looked forward to coming to therapy.

After several months of similar play, it shifted. Kirk began to use fantasy play that included larger and more varied toys and dress-up items. The familiar themes of aggression, victimization, danger, protection, rescue, and anxiety remained, but new themes emerged. At this point his play also reflected power and control, problem solving, and mastery. During this phase, he initially enacted fantasies involving police or military figures fighting some heinous crime. For several more months he began asserting himself through the play roles, and his behavior continued to improve in his foster home.

After 6 months of CCPT, Kirk began involving the therapist regularly in his imaginary play. He told the therapist that she was his wife; they were both police officers, with a family of two children. Kirk gave the therapist all the items she needed to keep herself and their babies safe, including guns, walkie-talkies, a knife, money, a telephone, a police hat, and a badge. Providing safety became a key theme for him.

While the therapist-as-wife cared for the children, Kirk left for his police job. He cuddled the children (dolls) and told his wife he loved her when he left. In one session, he told his wife to check for bullets around the house so that the babies would not find them. This play was repeated with some variations for many sessions, and the predominant theme of threat and safety continued, along with an emerging theme of family and relationships. Kirk was now 10 years old.

He began asking the therapist to come help him with the bad guys or hostage situations. He now took bows and arrows, handcuffs, and swords along with his helmet, badge, and guns. He also often put on armor to protect himself in the endless array of dangerous situations. He battled untold numbers of bad people, and most sessions ended when he arrested them with the help of his police officer wife (the therapist). He returned home to feed his children, often telling the babies, "Don't worry. You're safe!"

At this point, Kirk's sessions were interrupted by some placement difficulties. He was nearly adopted by his foster parents, and when they changed their minds, he began acting out once again. He was temporarily placed far away from the therapist. He returned to therapy when he was once again placed in a respite home in the therapist's region.

In the first CCPT session after his return, Kirk began with the police-couple play from prior sessions. This time, however, a rubber chicken attacked the babies, and he asked his wife (the therapist) to help him save the babies. There was lots of screaming and fighting with the chicken to save the children. When Kirk went off to his police job, he arrested two bad guys (large soft dolls), handcuffed them together, and threw them down. Kirk then staggered back to his wife, fell to the floor, and said, "They shot me." The therapist, in her wife role, grabbed the medical kit to help him. Kirk dramatically jerked and shook on the floor. The therapist joined the fantasy as expected: She took his blood pressure, gave him shots, and told Kirk that she would not let anything happen to him. He turned over onto his back and said, "They shot me in the heart." The therapist responded, "Oh, they broke your heart," and offered to put a Band-Aid on his heart (on top of his clothing).

He then got back up, returned to his prisoners, yelled at them, and told them he would go easy on them if they told the truth. He kept saying, "Don't lie to me. I'm the police, and you can't lie to me." After the session, the therapist wondered whether perhaps he was trying to make sense of the sudden loss of his foster family.

Kirk's CCPT play is interesting on several levels. Clearly, he now had a model of appropriate relationships and family caretaking. He felt safe and trusting enough to invite the therapist into his play, and he used the play to work on power, control, relationships, safety, danger, nurturance, and resilience themes. He was beginning to understand what healthy families were like, and that parents were responsible for the care and protection of children. He had begun to ask for help when he was afraid, and he felt more competent to address challenges and find solutions to problems.

When Kirk abruptly lost his foster family, he again felt powerless and afraid. Before therapy resumed, he had no support for those feelings and acted inappropriately. Decisions had been made in the foster care system that created further difficulties for him. He was confused and heartbroken. There was considerable regression in Kirk's real-world behavior during this unsettling time, but it stabilized as soon as the CCPT sessions began again. Therapy offered him the only stable relationship he had at the time.

Kirk eventually was placed with a new foster mother. She learned and conducted FT play sessions with him under the therapist's guidance, and his behavior settled more than it ever had. Kirk developed a healthy attachment relationship with the new mother and worked through considerably more of his trauma.

Perfectionism/Obsessive–Compulsive Disorder

Perfectionism and obsessive–compulsive disorder (OCD) are usually characterized by considerable anxiety. (Indeed, OCD is classified by the American Psychiatric Association [2000] as an anxiety disorder.) Perfectionistic or obsessive–compulsive behaviors are used to reduce this anxiety. CCPT can be helpful for children with these behaviors, because playfulness can offset some of the rigidity while releasing the anxiety. CCPT and FT have been conducted successfully with many perfectionistic children and families. Although children diagnosed with OCD may require additional treatment modalities, they often respond well to the nonjudgmental, noncritical climate of CCPT. Play sessions also offer them a new opportunity for control that is less disruptive and more adaptable.

Merilee was 11 years old. Her parents had divorced when she was 5; her father had remarried when she was 8; and her mother had recently begun a close relationship with a man from a nearby town. The mother and her new partner told the therapist during the intake that they were considering marriage, but wanted to move slowly so that Merilee could accept it. Merilee had been polite but reserved with the partner, telling her mother that he was nice but not as nice as her father.

Their primary complaint was Merilee's increasing perfectionism. She was in sixth grade and an excellent student. She spent at least 4 hours each night on homework that should have taken no more than 2 hours, according to her teacher. She also spent inordinate amounts of time with schoolwork on weekends. Merilee was also very sensitive to simple suggestions and seemed to think that everything was a criticism. Her father no longer lived in the area, but the therapist contacted him for his consent to treatment and input. He also reported anxious and perfectionistic tendencies in Merilee. He said she often spent much time selecting clothes to wear and applying nail polish. He and his wife often had to wait at least 20 extra minutes for her whenever they were going somewhere.

Merilee's mother admitted during the first meeting that she tended to be anxious, too, but not as intensely as Merilee. She was worried that Merilee was not happy and that her behaviors could worsen as she neared high school. Merilee presented as a rather serious girl, and during the family play observation with her mother, she chose to play "hangman" on the whiteboard for the entire time. In order to assess the situation further, the therapist suggested that she conduct a short course of CCPT before deciding to use FT and/or other interventions.

At first Merilee avoided most of the toys in the playroom. She commented that she preferred just to talk. The therapist responded, "You're not into these toys, and you're more comfortable talking about things. Well, in the special playroom, you can do just about anything you want, including talking, playing, or whatever." Merilee chose to play hangman with the therapist during the first session, and also told the therapist about her favorite school subjects. She was hesitant as she entered the playroom the second time. She walked around the room looking at the toys, and lingered in the section with dress-up clothes. She then played hangman again for a few minutes. She returned to the dress-up area, turned her back to the therapist, and tentatively put on a couple of hats. The therapist reflected in a warm tone of voice, "You're checking out a few other things. You're trying on a few hats to see what you look like in them." Merilee smiled at herself in the mirror when she put on a witch hat, and the therapist said, "You kinda like the witch look!"

Merilee warmed up a bit more during her third CCPT session. She immediately went to the dress-up clothing and put on the witch hat. She then put on a gaudy shawl and some fake green fingertips that had long bright red nails on them. She made faces at herself in the mirror. The therapist continued her empathic acceptance, saying, "Hey, you like that witch stuff. Now there's an outfit and those long red spiky nails. . . . It's fun for you to try out some different faces." At this, she turned to the therapist, squinted her eyes and frowned, raised her hands and curved her fingers to resemble claws, and cackled. She had transformed herself into a witch and was trying to scare the therapist. She was tacitly putting the therapist into a role, so the therapist acted scared: "Oh, no! There's a witch giving me the eye!" This brought laughter and relaxation. Merilee tried on several other outfits as her embarrassment diminished. She spent the entire session dressing and admiring herself in different costumes.

During her fourth session, Merilee told the therapist that they were going to play a game. The therapist was to be a school student, and Merilee would be the teacher. She dressed again in the witch outfit while the therapist sat at the small table with some crayons and papers. Merilee became the "evil teacher" who gave math questions to the student, corrected her papers, and wrote D's and F's in red crayon at the top of the papers. The therapist played the role of the exasperated student who tried hard but couldn't satisfy the teacher. Merilee loved this; she became more and more demanding as the teacher.

When they arrived for the next session, Merilee's mother said that she could see a small improvement: Merilee was spending more time at the dinner table before rushing off to do her homework. The therapist discussed possible sources of school-related anxiety with her mother, and the mother mentioned that when Merilee was in fourth grade, she had had a period of poor performance before they realized she needed glasses. It had not occurred to her mother that this might have started the spiral into excessive homework time.

Merilee continued to use the dress-up and fantasy play with the therapist to enact a number of themes related to school, authority, pleasing others, and making mistakes. She also continued to relax more at home. Because the therapist suspected some difficulties in Merilee's relationship with her mother, plans were made to begin FT sessions after the therapist had conducted 12 CCPT sessions with her. The CCPT and FT sessions alternated for a while before a complete shift to FT was made. As Merilee became increasingly playful, her mother realized that she had set a rather serious tone at home, and asked for suggestions on how she could become more playful herself. The therapist helped the two of them reconnect through play, and they had a warmer, more enjoyable relationship when they ended therapy.

Medical Illness

Medical illnesses in either children or parents cause worry and stress for families. This is especially true for chronic illnesses, such as diabetes, cancer, asthma, cystic fibrosis, and others. Chronic illnesses usually require changes in family lifestyle, unpleasant treatments, and complex medical management at home (VanFleet, 1986, 2000a). They are sometimes punctuated by more serious situations or hospitalizations that bring new worries. When children are thrust into the medical system through serious injury or chronic illness, their lives sometimes revolve around treatment or disease management, and they feel different from their peers. The boy in a body cast for multiple injuries sustained in a farm accident, the diabetic girl who must test her blood sugar levels with finger sticks and take several insulin injections daily, and the siblings visiting their mother who is in the hospital for cancer treatment all have something in common: Their lives are less in their control than if they did not have to contend with medical issues. For ill children, this loss of control can lead to medical compliance problems that propel families and medical professionals into a downward spiral, where increased emphasis on medical control leads to even more attempts by the children to resist that control. When parents are ill, they can lack the energy needed to attend to their children's needs as they wish, and behavioral problems can erupt.

CCPT and FT can be very useful tools for reestablishing some balance in these children and families. The play sessions provide ill children with a greater sense of control, so they are less likely to try to exert control in ways that interfere with their medical conditions. Play sessions also provide an opportunity for children to express their feelings about their own, their siblings', or their parents' illness. FT is a relatively short-term intervention that can bring families together in times of significant stress. Even parents feel more in control when they can do something positive to help their children cope with the situation.

Eleven-year-old Gayle had been in and out of the hospital her whole life. Both she and her older sister, Gina, had cystic fibrosis. Gina had recently died from the disease when she was 14. The therapist, a medical center psychologist and play therapist, had worked intermittently with the girls whenever they were hospitalized. (The family lived in a rural area 100 miles away.) The therapist had worked with Gayle and her sister together when it became clear that Gina was dying, and Gayle, who had loved horses from the time she was small, had told her sister before she died that heaven was probably full of horses.

The therapist, aware that Gayle probably had strong feelings about Gina's death as well as about the implications for her own illness and life, offered Gayle some additional CCPT sessions on her first hospitalization after her sister's death many months prior. Gayle had been refusing to eat sufficient quantities, and her body weight was dangerously low. This had been a chronic problem for both girls and had resulted in power struggles within the family. Gayle knew and liked the therapist, and immediately agreed to come to the playroom. Without hesitation, she pulled out all of the horses and placed them on a mat that she said was a field. The horses were playing, eating, and having a good time. The therapist commented, "Those horses are having a great time. They are playing and feeling good." Gayle then picked up a small bendable girl figure and said, "This is Gina." She placed the miniature Gina on top of one of the horses and moved them around, simulating a horse ride. The therapist reflected the feelings that Gayle's verbal and nonverbal behaviors indicated: "Gina really likes to ride. She's having a blast! Whoa! Gina almost fell off! Oh, she's doing tricks with the horse."

The therapist held six CCPT sessions with Gayle while she was in the hospital for that 2-week period. Gayle continued to use the horses to play out themes of loss, fear, hope, and health. The CCPT not only helped her with her feelings; it also seemed to redirect her control needs to her play, and her eating improved immediately. The therapist also used some directive interventions to hold a therapeutic funeral in the sandtray and to create a special book in honor of Gayle and Gina.

If the family had not lived so far away, FT would have been an excellent intervention to resolve the power struggles, to provide support for the parents, and to give Gayle an ongoing outlet for her worries.

Severe Trauma and Attachment Problems in Adolescents

CCPT is primarily used with children 3–12 years old—the ages when children use play and imagination most freely. When children have complex trauma coupled with attachment problems, however, their social and emotional development may be delayed. We have had experience using CCPT and FT with older children and adolescents under these circumstances, and have found that they find ways to use the play sessions for healing.

Liam was 13 years old when he was referred for therapy. He had just been released from a residential program that used outdoor experience as part of the treatment protocol. Liam had a history of physical, sexual, and emotional abuse; multiple placements and psychiatric hospitalizations; and numerous attachment disruptions. He had been removed from his family of origin at 6 years of age and moved within the child protective system at least 26 times. When the therapist told him that he "won the prize" for the most placements she ever heard of, and that he probably had learned ways to take care of himself, he immediately agreed with a hint of pride. Liam was a survivor. All of his energy seemed to focus on staying safe and preventing anyone from tricking him. He told the therapist that he had been to therapy many times before this, and that they were all the same. "All counselors ask the same stupid questions!" he said. He was resistant and presented with a tough manner. His physical appearance bore this stamp as well, with his long ponytail, T-shirt with cut-off sleeves, jeans whose waist rode so low most of his underwear showed, and temporary tattoos and ink drawings on his arms.

The therapist offered to show Liam the playroom, even though this seemed incongruent with his presentation. She was not sure what a boy like Liam would do in the playroom; he had already refused a snack she had offered at the start of the session. Liam entered the playroom and spent a long time looking over the toys. He picked up a few items that he thought were funny: a rubber chicken that squawks when it is squeezed, a fake cigarette, and a few hats and masks. He asked the therapist if he could wear the masks and take the chicken out to the waiting room to show his foster family. He seemed to be enjoying himself. He spent the remainder of the session trying to hit various targets with a soft dart gun. When the session was over, Liam said that he would like the snack now. He left smiling and agreed to come back to therapy. A relationship had begun.

When Liam arrived next time, he asked to go to the playroom. He also asked the therapist to make a video of him. He dressed in a pirate hat and covered his face with a black skeleton mask. He hid behind the large puppet theater and prepared some knives and swords. He told the therapist to begin filming, then came out from behind the theater. Without speaking, he immediately began pretending that he was being assaulted by a huge stuffed bear and an equally large purple stuffed dinosaur with jagged teeth. As he enacted the scene, the bear and the dinosaur took turns attacking Liam. Often he was on the floor with the attacker on top of him. Each time he was attacked, he fought back fiercely; he was animated and dramatic. Each time he began to get up in victory, one of the animals attacked him again. At one point he pretended that his foes were banging his head against the wall, when he was using his fists to make the noise (out of sight). He grunted and groaned as the battle wore on. Liam continued the intense and energetic fight for 10 minutes, never speaking. In the play, one of his attackers stabbed him, and he died dramatically with the sword held between his arm and his side. He wore the mask throughout. He ended the action scene, told the therapist he wanted to see the video of his work, and left the playroom appearing calm and happy.

The therapist, using empathic listening, narrated his play by using feeling and intention reflections and tracking the action. Liam did not object to this. The empathic listening responses centered on how hard Liam had to fight for his life; how tired he had become from the battle; how each time he thought he had won and it was over, the enemies managed to rise again and come after him; and how there was danger lurking everywhere, with no safe place for Liam to go. According to Liam's records, this was certainly similar to his life experience. His parents had made money for drugs by offering him and his siblings to sexual predators. He later told the therapist that he had felt responsible for his brothers' safety and had cared for them the best he could.

At this early stage, however, Liam had no intention of talking with the therapist about his history. He guarded his privacy and had little trust in a system that had hurt him many times. He saw the therapist as part of that system. He resented the decisions made for him without his input or knowledge, and he had accumulated much anger. Offering Liam a wide variety of materials and the opportunity to work in a way of his own choosing seemed to open the door. The dramatic play offered a window into Liam's world. His hypervigilance and distancing made sense for a person who had experienced such danger. The aggression in his play seemed to be a way of protecting himself and staying safe, symbolically fighting for his life. Perhaps his most notable theme during CCPT sessions was his resilience: No matter what happened, he fought back bravely. Other play themes were aggression, danger, protection, evil, power, control, and lack of trust in the environment.

In Liam's third session, he chose large soft dolls to do a puppet show. This time he asked the therapist to observe the show while he gave voice to the characters. Liam had an active sense of humor, so much of the show featured the squawking chicken pecking and harassing the other characters. The others were afraid of the chicken, which kept reappearing to its own musical theme, sung by Liam in a manner reminiscent of the well-known bass notes signaling the appearance of the shark in the movie Jaws.

In Liam's scenario, the three primary characters were in similar situations, being harassed by the chicken and trying to overcome hardships thrown upon them. One of the characters, a boy doll, seemed kind and gentle. This boy character met a cute little bunny, whom he addressed politely; the bunny surprised the boy by biting him in the face. The boy was surprised and confused by the bunny's hurtful behavior. He told the bunny that he did not appreciate his behavior, but the bunny laughed and did not seem to care. The boy told another imaginary character of his plight, and that character spoke rudely and rejected him. Finally, the boy doll was thrown out of the theater entirely. He found no one to listen or have sympathy for him. The meanest character then tossed all the others out of the "house" and said, "I'm the coolest one around."

In this expressive and dramatic play, it seemed that the boy character was trying to find someone to trust, but met with failure. The distinct theme was one of asking for help, only to be ignored, discarded, and hurt again. This appeared to be a rather hopeless situation, unless, of course, a character could be stronger and meaner than all the others. That was the only way to stay safe and avoid being hurt. The theme of Liam's play seemed symbolic of his actual life.

Liam had much therapeutic work to do. The CCPT sessions opened the door for this resistant adolescent to form a relationship with the therapist and begin that work. At the end of these three sessions, Liam told the therapist that no other therapy setting had been as "cool" as this one. No others had toys or snacks. He decided to talk with his guardian ad litem and ask to come to therapy twice a week. The request was granted by the court, because Liam had never before shown such interest and initiative in any prior therapeutic experiences. The safety of CCPT engaged Liam, and he was motivated to begin his healing journey.

Acute Trauma

Tyrone was 3 years old when referred for treatment by his pediatrician. He had witnessed his 6-month-old baby sister's being bitten all over her face and body by a 2-year-old child in their day care setting. The care provider had stepped outside for a telephone call when the other child victimized the baby. Tyrone had tried to protect his sister, then called for help, but no adults were available to stop the attack. Tyrone told his mother that he was upset because he could not stop it. The baby was severely injured and required follow-up medical care for months. The same child had bitten Tyrone once in the past, and the day care provider had accused Tyrone of provoking that attack. This made it difficult for Tyrone to comprehend the current event.

Tyrone's parents described him as a happy, talkative, and bright boy prior to the attack on his sister. After the incident, he had many toileting "accidents," frequent vomiting, and disturbed sleep patterns. He also became more withdrawn, as well as obsessed with "messes" that he felt compelled to clean up.

The family was close-knit. The children and their parents enjoyed each other's company and played together often. The parents were eager for help, so that Tyrone would not be saddled with a lifetime of unresolved trauma. Tyrone had been at this day care setting for a long time, and he felt close to the woman who ran it. When his parents, fearing for their children's safety, immediately removed them from the day care center, Tyrone's trauma reactions were compounded by the loss of the relationship with his provider and the disruption in his daily routine.

Tyrone first saw the playroom when he came with his parents for a family play observation during the assessment phase. He was a bit shy with the therapist, but eager to enter the playroom. After he played with his parents for 20 minutes, they sat in the corner behind a desk and observed as the therapist held a CCPT session with Tyrone. Tyrone's play involved cleaning up the "filth." His mother laughed as Tyrone commented on all the "messes," and how important it was to clean them up. When his mother heard Tyrone say he had to stay on top of all the messes, she wondered whether Tyrone was mimicking things she herself had said at home. She later told the therapist that she would now be more aware of how often she said such things.

Because the therapeutic plan was to move quickly into FT, the mother observed from the corner again. Play themes during this CCPT session centered on being good, taking care of a baby sister character, and playroom exploration.

A third CCPT session was held with the mother observing. Tyrone played intensely during this session. His primary themes were of danger, protection, power, control, and safety. In his play, Tyrone cared for a baby—thoughtfully dressing and feeding it, and making sure the baby had everything it needed. He was very nurturing. He then selected several stuffed animals that had big teeth and placed them on the floor while he saw to the baby's safety. As he guarded the baby doll, he yelled at the animals and threw things at them. He announced that no animals with big teeth could hurt the baby. He shouted that they were never to return again. He was intense and very engaged throughout this sequence. At the end of the session, he left without hesitation, and he appeared calm, relaxed, and happy.

After this session, the mother reported that Tyrone was functioning much better. He had started at a new day care center without problems; he was sleeping through the night; and his digestive and toileting troubles subsided. Because of this seemingly rapid resolution to his trauma reactions, the therapist held just two more CCPT sessions. Here Tyrone played briefly with the doll and then painted. He seemed content, and his parents reported that his improvements at home continued. It appeared that Tyrone had managed to gain control over the negative impact this unfortunate and frightening incident had had on him. His pretrauma level of well-being had been restored. The therapist offered to conduct FT with the parents at any time in the future that they wished.

Oppositional Defiant Disorder

Marvin, 4 years old, was brought to therapy by his parents. His mother had been diagnosed with cancer and had undergone treatments in a city far from their home. She had stayed with relatives in the city and returned home intermittently, but she had been largely unavailable during the preceding 18 months. Marvin's father had to work longer hours to pay for medical bills that were not covered by their insurance, so Marvin and his 6-year-old brother had often stayed with their aunt during their mother's absence. Marvin was the identified client because of his behavior pattern, which resembled oppositional defiant disorder (ODD), although it had not been formally diagnosed as such. He had become extremely hard to manage, and he resisted most requests that his parents made. His mother, Anne, was in remission and feeling much better, and she was living at home again. His father, Chris, was still working long hours. His older brother, Roger, was not viewed as a problem.

Anne and Chris told the therapist that they had expected Marvin's behavior to improve once his mother returned home, but it did not. Marvin was particularly oppositional with Chris, who said he had felt guilty about disciplining Marvin when he was missing his mother while she was away. The parents described several battles every day with Marvin over such things as going to bed, getting up, brushing his teeth, watching television, putting his toys away, coming for meals, and using the bathroom. Whatever they requested, Marvin resisted. His resistance came in the form of ignoring, talking back ("NO!"), insulting them ("You're a bad mommy!"), whining, crying, throwing tantrums, holding his breath, and literally digging in his heels. There seemed no end to his creativity in finding ways to oppose them. They tried to ignore him, but he wore them down. They tried time outs, but he outlasted them. Things had been getting worse rather than better since Anne's return home.

During the assessment, which included a family play observation, the therapist noted that much of the family energy surrounded Marvin. Roger stayed on the periphery and seemed eager to keep everyone happy. He quickly relinquished his toys to Marvin in order to prevent conflict. Although the parents did not see problems with Roger, the therapist was concerned that he might be depressed. The therapist recommended FT, to be used with both boys. Both parents participated in the training phase and quickly learned the special play session skills. They then took turns holding one-to-one play sessions with each of the boys.

Roger was hesitant at first, but his play became more expansive within just a few sessions. The more he played, the more he relaxed. Having the special times alternately with his parents seemed to give him some of the attention and acceptance he really needed. His depressive demeanor lifted quickly, especially after he did some attachment play with his mother, in which he handcuffed her to him so that she wouldn't get "lost in the forest."

At first Marvin's play did not resemble that of typical 4-year-olds. He carefully organized the smallest miniatures in the playroom, and he separated small guns and weapons into piles. His mother told the therapist that he slept with a toy gun under his pillow.

Marvin occasionally broke the playroom rules, and his parents improved in their abilities to set limits with him. The therapist had educated them about oppositionality, noting in particular that it was often driven by anxiety. They discussed how the many changes during the past year and a half had created anxiety for Marvin, and how his misbehaviors and obsessively oppositional patterns were his misguided attempts to regain control. The therapist, based on much prior experience with children who had ODD, believed that shifting Marvin's control to the playroom would reduce his need for control over all household decisions. Marvin thoroughly enjoyed the play sessions with his parents, and for the most part was not oppositional during them. He sometimes resisted leaving the playroom, however. During one session, his father had to take him by the hand and gently lead him out into the waiting area, where he then had a tantrum.

Anne and Chris mastered the play session skills and were ready to start their home play sessions after 5 weeks of live supervision by the therapist. Marvin was eager for this and asked daily when his play sessions would be held. The therapist met with the parents regularly to discuss the home sessions. During his second home session with Chris, Marvin defiantly broke a rule three times, necessitating the end of the play session. The following week as their next play session began, he told his father, "Tell me when it's time to leave. I might forget. Tell me. Tell me." This signaled his desire to be compliant and an awareness that he could not do it on his own. In his play session with Anne that week, he played a game of hide and seek, during which he laughed heartily for the first time in months. His organizing of miniatures gave way to more typical active play for his age, and his play themes reflected aggression, power, control, mastery, and relationship building. His parents reported that he thoroughly enjoyed the sessions, as did they.

After a total of 11 play sessions, Marvin's daily ODD-like behaviors were gone. The control he exerted in the playroom was more appropriately placed, and the play sessions with his parents' balanced and consistent use of acceptance and boundaries added to his sense of security.

Roger's play throughout the process was quieter, but he enjoyed it thoroughly as well. He often created roads in the sandbox and ran cars over them, surmounting obstacles that were in the way. He seemed to be doing the same in daily life. In one session, he asked Anne whether he could tip over a small table that had paper and some markers on it. She reflected and said he could do just about anything. In slow motion, he tipped it over so that the markers and paper were scattered on the floor and the table was upended. He stepped back, folded his arms, and with a satisfied look on his face stated, "Wow. Wait till Daddy sees this disaster!" This tiny sign of "naughtiness" was seen as a positive sign that Roger was relaxing and allowing himself to be a boy, rather than trying to be perfect at all times. He began to assert himself a bit more within the family and seemed to enjoy things more than he had.

Anne and Chris successfully generalized their use of the skills to daily life, and the family ended formal therapy after a total of 17 sessions. They continued holding special playtimes at home, and they told the therapist in a telephone conversation a year later that the improvements had been maintained.

Summary

The case vignettes outlined here are by no means exhaustive of the possible applications of CCPT, but they provide illustrations of what this approach looks like in action. Both children with mild, transitory problems and children with complex, entrenched difficulties frequently benefit from CCPT (used either alone or in conjunction with other interventions). Once children realize that the freedom to choose their own path through play is real, they often move quickly into themes that are symbolic of their feelings and circumstances. Children must feel safe in order to play freely, and CCPT offers a unique safety that is both accepting and healing. Children tend to embrace it readily when it is conducted properly by therapists or by parents under the supervision of an FT therapist.

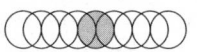

CHAPTER 10

Handling Select Child Behaviors and Special Circumstances

Children react and behave in different ways during nondirective play sessions, and therapists must be prepared to apply the skills and principles of CCPT flexibly in a variety of unpredictable situations. Furthermore, because CCPT sessions give children greater choice and leeway than is possible or desirable in daily life, therapists must make decisions about behaviors that normally are not encouraged or permitted. This chapter covers ways to handle some of the child behaviors and feelings that nondirective play therapists encounter, and that tend to be handled differently than in daily life or even in other forms of therapy.

Bossiness

Some children take full advantage of the permissive atmosphere of CCPT sessions, and they create roles for themselves of power and domination. At times they create roles where they are the authority or "boss," such as parent, teacher, police officer, villain, hero, or monster. They can become quite bossy in these roles, demanding that the therapist, in his or her imaginary role, perform a variety of acts that on the surface may seem diminishing or demeaning.

Valerie was a 10-year-old girl who had a history of abuse and many placements within the foster care system. Although she was bright, she did poorly in school because of the interference of her emotional reactions to events, especially unexpected ones. Valerie immediately engaged with CCPT, and her enthusiasm for the play sessions was clear. She quickly grasped the idea that she had much more power and control than in real life, and by the second session, she assumed a variety of roles where she was in charge. In the fifth session, she pretended she was a teacher, with several large dolls serving as her students. She wrote on the blackboard, periodically turning to the members of her "class" and correcting their behavior: "I told you to shut up! Now do what I say!" Before long, she turned to the therapist and told her to sit next to the dolls; she was to be a student as well. The therapist entered the imaginary role of student. Valerie then focused most of her attention on her live student, telling her words to spell and math problems to solve. Valerie then took the papers, corrected them with a large red crayon, and returned them to her student for more work. She told the therapist-as-student that she was stupid and sneaky, and that if she (as the teacher) caught her cheating, there would be big problems. Of course, she created a situation where she claimed the student was cheating, and she began yelling, "You are nothin'! You don't know squat. You are stupid, stupid, *stupid*! Grow up and shut up. Do 100 more spelling words! You're never gonna get it right!" The therapist played the role of a confused, inadequate student, as seemed to be Valerie's intent.

This example shows bossy language and behavior that most people would find disturbing if it occurred in daily life situations. This was Valerie's therapy, however, and the therapist handled it appropriately, following Valerie's lead in how she played the assigned role. On the surface, one might worry that the therapist was reinforcing undesirable behavior, but Valerie's bossy play was clearly done in an imaginative manner that suggested she was expressing some of her feelings about her life in general and school in particular. When children play bossy or demanding roles, they are more likely to be sharing some of their feelings of frustration or inadequacy, rather than any intention to become social pariahs.

Perhaps the primary message of this chapter is that for therapists to truly understand children and their play behaviors, they must look beyond the surface or literal behaviors to the broader or more symbolic meanings of the play *for the children*. In a literal sense, Valerie's play was rude and demanding; yet when the therapist told her the session was over, Valerie immediately dropped her bossy demeanor and complied with the therapist, leaving the playroom. She was polite and respectful. This sudden change to socially appropriate behavior clearly indicates that her bossiness was contained within the imaginary role of teacher.

Was Valerie revealing a disturbed hidden self with intention to dominate and disrespect adults? Probably not. In fact, Valerie had difficulty in school and felt she could never please her teachers; her play seemed more indicative of that dynamic. Considered in context, it seemed more likely that Valerie cast her therapist in her own real-life school role while she tested out the more powerful and attractive role of teacher. Perhaps she was both (1) communicating her damaged feelings of self-worth at school (how she made her therapist-as-student feel), and (2) experimenting with feelings of greater power and control. Had her therapist not played along with Valerie's assigned roles as she did, this important communication and therapeutic work might have been thwarted.

When therapists view children's play too literally, they risk missing the real message or intent of the play. Furthermore, when therapists begin to consider more adult reactions and interpretations of children's play during play sessions, they are no longer attending to or empathizing fully with the children's perspectives, and they fail to be wholly accepting of children's needs and expressions at that point.

Bad Words

Adults also often become concerned with children's behavior when children say what the adults consider "bad words." In CCPT, therapists typically permit children to say anything during the session, including bad words. The words themselves can do no actual harm, and they are expressions of feelings or attitudes, or forms of experimentation. Because most children understand that play sessions offer greater freedom than daily life, it is unlikely that this practice actually creates or worsens real-life behavior.

Why do children use bad words? It can reflect their natural curiosity as they learn about taboo expressions. It can be a method to provoke adult reactions, especially if parents and teachers have acted shocked and alarmed, thereby reinforcing the behavior. It can stem from the reinforcement they have received when peers have giggled at the forbidden expressions. Finally, some children may routinely hear these expressions from the adults in their lives and may be imitating them.

Handling bad words is another area in which CCPT therapists must be aware of their own internal reactions, so they can keep what they are feeling and thinking congruent with their in-session behavior. It is desirable for therapists to be comfortable enough to hear and *accept* children's expressions. For example, when a child says, "Shit!" when he or she can't get a toy to work, the therapist reflects the child's feeling: "It's frustrating—you're having trouble getting that to work." If a child looks knowingly at the therapist while saying, "Damn, damn, damn, shit, shit, stupid-head," the therapist might respond, "You like being able to say those words," or even "You really think it's funny to say 'damn' and 'shit' and 'stupid-head'—words you usually aren't allowed to say." This level of acceptance frequently surprises children, and often such forays into foul language are short-lived. Bad words are often used in situations where children are working through their powerlessness by behaving powerfully.

The key here, as always, is to consider each child's behavior—including verbalizations—in context to determine its meaning for the child. Doing this will help the therapist determine the most accurate and attuned response. Sometimes there are surprises, as the following exchange with a 7-year-old girl during a CCPT session illustrates.

GIRL: Do you know any bad words?

THERAPIST: Sounds like you're thinking about bad words.

GIRL: Uh-huh. Do you know any?

THERAPIST: You're really curious about those words.

GIRL: I know the F-word!

THERAPIST: You're excited to know the F-word!

GIRL: (*Giggling and whispering*) Fart!

THERAPIST: You think that's very funny.

For many reasons, it is important for therapists to withhold their judgment and to be accepting when they encounter bad words.

When children are angry, they can say unkind or even vicious words or try to provoke a reaction from the therapist, to test the therapist's level of true acceptance. For example, a novice play therapist sought supervision over a 10-year-old girl who frequently called the therapist such names as "inept shrink," "loser," or "idiot." During supervision, this therapist came to realize that this child was tapping into the therapist's own vulnerabilities, as she had been raised by a very emotionally abusive mother herself. With this recognition, and armed with some reflective responses to use with this child, the therapist was able to regain her accepting stance. The therapist was better able to reach the depth of the child's feelings by accurately reflecting them: "You're angry and like to try to hurt with your words," and "You're disappointed in me and don't like how I am being with you." Much to the novice therapist's surprise, reaching the depth of this child's feelings allowed the child to feel understood and accepted. The child no longer had to resort to name calling. She had been heard. In fact, the child admitted to the thera- pist that she didn't believe anyone really could like her, so she "tested" people by calling them the worst names to see whether her words would end her relationships with them. When a child says hurtful things to a therapist, it is rarely actually *about* the therapist. Such verbal behaviors convey much more about the child's distress, and when the therapist can be accepting at the deepest levels, the child is more likely to work through the core problems in a therapeutic climate of acceptance.

Although it is important for therapists to become as accepting as possible of children's use of foul or unkind language, there are sometimes phrases or words that individual therapists may not be able to tolerate. For example, a devoutly religious therapist may find some expressions unacceptable, or a therapist who is a member of a racial minority group may find it difficult to accept children who make derogatory racial slurs. When a therapist simply cannot bear to hear some bad words, it is bet- ter for him or her to set a limit on those particular words or phrases. For example, an overweight therapist might say, "Celia, one of the things you cannot do in here is to call me a 'fatty,' but you can do and say almost anything else." To be clear under these circumstances, the thera- pist should actually tell the child the word or phrase that is forbidden in a neutral, matter-of-fact manner. It is important to minimize the num- ber of limits set around children's verbal expressions, so as not to restrict avenues of communication and healing unnecessarily, and to be as fully accepting of children as possible.

A case example of FT illustrates how acceptance of bad words helped alter a boy's relationship with his mother. Ten-year-old Nathan came to therapy with his mother because of problems with his opposi- tional behavior and angry feelings, which were out of control at home. He was a high achiever; there was considerable family pressure to excel in academics and sports; and his oppositional behavior seemed under- girded by anxiety. His relationship with his mother was very strained. After she had been trained in the play session skills and was antici- pating her first session with Nathan, the mother anxiously asked the therapist what she should do if he cursed. The therapist told her that he was likely to curse if that was a concern of hers. The therapist then suggested ways the mother could respond in an accepting manner, using the nondirective play skills.

As anticipated, Nathan immediately tested his mother by playing aggressive themes and cursing. He said that he was a pirate, and when he cursed as part of that role, his mother empathically listened: "You really like saying those words that you are not allowed to say outside of the playroom. You're checking to see how I'm reacting to that." Nathan laughed and said a few more words. It appeared that his cursing vocabulary was very limited, and that he had exhausted the words he knew in a few seconds. His mother's reflection had conveyed her acceptance of this behavior during the play sessions, and it seemed to establish emotional safety for him to use the playroom as he needed. At this point he told his mother that she was a pirate, too, and then he pretended to shoot her. His mother "died" dramatically, playing the role as she thought he wished. He laughed and looked at the therapist in disbelief that his mother had actually enacted the death scene as a pirate. From that point on, he frequently invited his mother to join his imaginary play, and his cursing and testing behaviors decreased quickly. The enjoyment shared by Nathan and his mother resulted in relatively quick improvements in their relationship.

Cheating

During CCPT sessions, it is quite common for children to play games or create competitive activities that give themselves the advantage. For example, an 8-year-old boy invited his therapist to play a ring-toss game with him. He told the therapist to stand about 8 feet away from the target post, while he stood only 2 feet away. It was clearly much easier for him to succeed than for the therapist.

Adults often refer to this type of behavior as "cheating" and try to teach children to "play fair." In a ring-toss game in real life, for instance, most adults would insist that all the players toss their rings from the same distance. This is handled differently in CCPT, and closer examination of the situation in this example from the child's point of view reveals that it might not have been cheating at all! The boy was competing with an adult who was taller, with longer arms and more experience. After all, the therapist was the owner of the ring-toss game! The boy could have considered these qualities to be unfair advantages and might simply have been rearranging the rules to "even the playing field."

Furthermore, it is useful to consider other reasons *why* children cheat. Unless children don't understand the rules of the game, cheating behaviors usually reflect children's lack of confidence. Some children, for a variety of reasons, have a strong need to win. Losing is intolerable for them, and they may have difficulty in their relationships with siblings or peers because of this. In this case, being able to play the winner's role relates directly to their problem. In CCPT, the therapist would acknowledge the need and the role: "You really wanted to win, and it feels great to be the champion." Related to this, some children realize that they lack the skill to have any chance of winning if they must play by the usual rules. When they obviously alter the rules to their own advantage, the therapist might respond, "You want to make *sure* that you can win this game. It's very important to you."

What typically happens in CCPT is that children play with a "loaded deck" for a few sessions. As their skill and/or confidence develops, they reduce the unevenness of the competition. Janice, at 11, had few friends because of her unrelenting need to win any game. There was considerable pressure on her from her family to excel in all things she tried. She was increasingly anxious about school or any skill-based activities. The therapist used several modalities in working with the family, but Janice's problems surfaced early in her CCPT sessions. She asked the therapist to play the card game War, with her. During the first three games of War, spanning three sessions, Janice pulled out the four aces before shuffling the cards and kept them for herself, thereby assuring an eventual victory. During the fourth game of War in a subsequent session, Janice pulled only two aces for herself, and in the next game she shuffled the deck without extracting any aces. Janice now seemed more comfortable playing within the rules. This process occurs commonly in children who cheat during their play sessions and is a manifestation of increased self-esteem. Their self-worth is no longer tied to winning all the time and at any cost.

Very Withdrawn Behaviors

Some children have separation anxiety or exhibit very withdrawn behaviors with the therapist during their first CCPT sessions. When a child refuses to leave a parent or other accompanying adult, the therapist can invite the adult to sit near the playroom door where the child can see him or her. The therapist can structure the situation by giving the adult some paper to write down any questions or concerns, and then offers the child the playroom. The therapist should reflect the child's feelings of anxiety: "You're not too sure about me and this situation. It's pretty strange to you, and you're worried. Your mom [dad, etc.] is going to sit right here, and I'm going to show you our special playroom. It's a place where you can do just about anything you want, and if there's something you can't do, I'll let you know." Some withdrawn children respond well at this point, while others remain withdrawn.

At this point, the therapist assumes a nonthreatening posture, sitting or kneeling on the floor, usually at some distance from the child. In a matter-of-fact and friendly tone, the therapist continues to reflect the child's feelings: "This is pretty new to you, and you're just not sure about it at all. You're checking things out, but it feels scary right now. You're not sure what to do. You really can do just about anything in here." When the child is silent, the therapist slows the pacing of these statements, but continues to focus on the child's feelings. If direct eye contact makes the child uneasy, the therapist avoids it. The key is to create a safe and accepting environment, and this is done by tuning in to the child's nonverbal signals and by providing accepting empathic statements.

Only in extreme cases where the child seems at risk of being traumatized by the experience would the therapist attempt a further intervention. A fairly benign and mostly nondirective intervention would be to pick up a puppet and make the empathic and structuring statements through that. Tonnie, a 3-year-old girl in kinship care with her grandmother, refused to leave her grandmother's side. She clung to her grandmother's dress just inside the playroom door. The grandmother encouraged her to look around and then, following the therapist's instructions, permitted the therapist to handle the situation from there. Tonnie quickly hid under an easel that was nearby. After several minutes of calm, quiet reflections, the therapist picked up a small lamb puppet. Using a higher-pitched voice as the lamb, the therapist said, "Hey, Tonnie, I can see that this place is kinda scary for you. But that lady is right—you can play with all these toys and do just about anything that you want." Slowly, Tonnie peeked from the bottom edge of the easel. She hesitantly rolled a ball across the floor, and the lamb responded, "Hey, Tonnie, I see that you rolled out that ball. You're waiting to see what will happen." Before long, Tonnie began playing with more of the toys, and the therapist resumed the empathic listening as herself.

If this type of intervention has no impact, and the child continues to show signs of terror or traumatization, the therapist might introduce a more directive activity in order to establish sufficient emotional safety for the child. This should be done only in the most extreme cases, as it violates the Axlinian principles of letting children lead the way and solve their own problems. In this case, the therapist offers a "tour" of the playroom—walking around with the child and adult, showing them the various toys, and demonstrating how they work (in a minimal way). The therapist should make sure to touch the many different types of toys and to avoid suggesting any particular toy for the child to play with. As quickly as possible, the therapist resumes the CCPT process by reiterating the room entry statement.

Therapists must evaluate carefully their own desire to "rescue" children from their anxiety. It is often likely that a child's anxiety is the reason for referral, and a therapist does not wish to give a less-than-empowering message by offering too much caretaking. Usually empathic listening statements are sufficient encouragement for withdrawn children to begin looking around the room. The therapist accepts their feelings and gives them time to overcome their own anxieties. Sometimes it can take several sessions of quiet and minimal exploration before such children begin to play more freely. The more active interventions are used *only* when children's anxiety rises to extreme levels, and in order to prevent creating a traumatic association with the playroom. If children are merely quiet and avoidant, the therapist continues to follow the usual CCPT process without further intervention until they feel safer.

Aggression

Many therapists are concerned about children's aggressive play themes and behaviors. It is helpful to make a distinction between *real* aggression (behaviors that could result in actual injury or destruction) and *imaginary* aggression (behaviors that are more reflective of children's feelings and issues). In general, CCPT therapists set limits on the former and are accepting of the latter. This is a more complex matter than this simple statement suggests, however.

Aggressive play is common. Many animal species engage in play fighting, which is distinguished from real fighting by various communication signals. For example, dogs frequently engage in play fighting, signaling their intent in various ways (e.g., the playful crouch known as a "play bow," ears pricked forward, and tails in a relaxed wag). These gestures and expressions are absent or very different during real fighting. In many ways, children do the same type of signaling, with facial expressions, gestures, and "Let's pretend . . . " or similar words. Children's play fighting is common and normal (Jones, 2002; Mechling, 2008), although it can sometimes cross boundaries into real antagonism, and these are the instances where adult supervision helps contain it. One of the challenges of childhood is learning how to handle normal aggressive impulses and how to channel them in prosocial ways. Children need opportunities for imaginary aggressive play in order to learn this. Jones (2002) offers a thought-provoking exploration of this topic. It is common in play therapy for children to exhibit aggressive play themes, and it is important for therapists to understand them and how to respond to them.

In an early comprehensive study of FT, B. G. Guerney and Stover (1971) found that aggressive play occurred early in CCPT, usually in sessions immediately after the exploratory play of the first session or two. It peaked and then diminished, but never disappeared entirely. In our own experience, this same pattern has emerged consistently.

There are two key factors in therapists' handling of aggressive behaviors in children. The first is to determine when limits should be set and when simply to reflect or engage in assigned imaginary play roles. The second is to ensure a high level of skill when responding to children's aggressive play.

To Listen or to Limit?

Although therapists have individual variations and tolerance levels for aggressive play behaviors, a general rule follows: If any behavior could imminently result in injury to a child, injury to a therapist, mass destruction of toys, or destruction of valuable toys, the therapist should set a limit on this behavior and enforce this limit firmly. Doing so is important for physical and emotional safety. For example, if a child is having a sword fight, and the sword swings within a few inches of the therapist's face, the therapist should set a limit, perhaps on how close the sword can come. If a child starts to eat some Play-Doh (with a real consequence of illness likely), the therapist would set a limit. If a child uses a sharp object to try to puncture the bop bag, it is time for a limit. If a child asks the therapist to spank him or her "for real," the therapist refuses by establishing a limit on actual hitting of other people.

On the other hand, when the play behavior is not likely to result in any real-time injury or major destruction, the therapist aims to be accepting of it by listening empathically or by playing any assigned role related to it. For example, if the child stabs a doll in an effort to kill it, the therapist listens empathically. If a child tells the therapist to pretend that he or she is a witch who casts evil spells and turns children into dragons, the therapist cackles in a witch-like manner and dramatically points a finger at the child, saying, "Heh, heh, heh, you are now a *dragon!*" If the child points an unloaded gun (no actual projectiles) at the therapist and pretends to shoot, the therapist enacts a death scene, coming back to life on the child's command or when the child moves to other play. If the child pretends to have a miniature father figure beat up a miniature mother figure, the therapist responds, "That guy is really hurting that woman." It is important for the therapist to remember that this *is* the child's actual therapeutic work taking place, and that acceptance of it is critical. Anything less is likely to shut down the child's communication and therapeutic work on this critical area.

Ensuring High-Level Skilled Responses

Almost always, children's aggressive play is not merely about violence and aggression. A surface behavior may be aggressive, but its meaning for a child goes deeper. If one believes, as CCPT therapists do, that children's play represents their inner worlds and perceptions, and that they work through problems by means of their play, then it is desirable to permit them to play out any themes that do not require limits. Often it appears that children who play aggressively may actually feel vulnerable in daily life. Given the opportunity to play as they wish, they choose themes of power and control to counteract the vulnerability or anxiety or fearfulness they experience in daily life. For example, an 8-year-old boy was referred to a play therapist after uncharacteristically threatening to "beat up" some of his classmates. His father had recently separated from his mother and had told him, "Now you are the man of the family." In actuality, the boy was frightened of his new "responsibilities," knowing full well that he was a vulnerable child attempting to take on a confusing adult role. In his play sessions, the boy engaged in aggressive play themes at first, such as when the mother doll fought with the father doll and threw him off the roof of the house. He also had to vanquish the "bad guys" on numerous occasions, using many weapons to do so. The more that he played this way, the fewer problems were reported by his mother and teachers. It seemed that he was able to feel safer and more powerful in the play sessions, and the need to gain power with his peers was diminished.

If play therapists reflect only children's aggressive or violent feelings and play content, then they are missing the deeper meanings of the play. To help children work through their own difficulties with aggression, power, and control, CCPT therapists look for the more fundamental feelings *beneath* the aggressive play. Frequently the underlying feelings include the following:

- Anger
- Frustration
- Vulnerability
- Insecurity
- Need for greater safety
- Helplessness
- Power and control
- "Can you accept me and all my feelings?" (an unspoken question for the therapist)
- "Can you contain me and keep me safe?" (another unspoken question)
- Communications of how the child has felt in daily life

In addition, sometimes the play is a reenactment of abuse or domestic violence, and shame or guilt is attached to the undisclosed experience. It is particularly important for therapists to be accepting of the aggression in such cases, so that they can eventually reach the shameful feelings that need to be resolved for healing to occur.

Skillful therapist responses start with reflections of children's aggressive themes and feelings, but then move to the underlying feelings. This helps children feel accepted and allows them to continue to resolve the fears and anxieties that are fueling the aggressiveness. An example follows.

Nine-year-old Leslie pretended she was a witch who cast evil spells on children (dolls). In daily life, she had been arguing with her newly adopted younger sister. Leslie had also been physically abused by one of her mother's boyfriends when she was 6 years old.

LESLIE: I'm the evil witch, and I'm going to chop the babies' heads off! (*Cackles.*)

THERAPIST: Ooooh! You are going to chop off their heads.

LESLIE: (*Laughing*) Yeah! Watch this. (*Pretends to chop off a head with her sword.*)

THERAPIST: There goes one head. That baby is a goner. You really wanted to get rid of her.

LESLIE: Yeah! She was bad, bad, bad. She was eeeevil. (*Chops off another head.*)

THERAPIST: There goes another one. You need to get rid of those bad ones before they can cause trouble.

LESLIE: They already caused trouble. That's all they do is cause trouble!

THERAPIST: The trouble sounds awful. You want to make sure there's no more. It feels good to get rid of all those problems. Whew! What a relief—no more trouble!

LESLIE: Now I'm going to be a princess. (*Dresses herself up as a princess.*)

THERAPIST: Now you're the princess with a crown and lots of jewelry.

LESLIE: I'm going to teach the bad babies some manners in princess school.

THERAPIST: You're going to try to help them stop causing all that trouble.

In this example, the therapist eventually reflected the child's feelings about how awful the trouble felt and her desire to eliminate it. Leslie was then able to shift to an alternative way of resolving her symbolic dilemma.

Aggressive play seems to generate more questions and concerns from novice CCPT therapists than almost any other type of play. This is probably because they are reacting to the surface components of the play without considering the underlying feelings and dynamics. When therapists recognize and accept the more fundamental feelings beneath the aggression, such as powerlessness, hurt, or fear, children feel understood and empowered to solve their own challenges. Of course, therapists have their own limitations and sensitivities about certain types of play, and they must set limits on behaviors where they do not feel safe. On the other hand, if therapists are uncomfortable with most aggressive play, they can increase their tolerance through training and supervision. Usually, when therapists gain more confidence in their limit-setting abilities, they are ready to be more accepting of the imaginary aggressive play that represents a child's inner world and dilemmas. The balance between setting limits on actual aggression and accepting imaginary aggression is crucial for the child's eventual resolution of aggression and the anxieties that underlie it.

Does Acceptance in CCPT Open Pandora's Box in Daily Life?

Novice play therapists sometimes wonder whether permitting certain behaviors in the playroom can cause increases in those behaviors in daily life. The answer is "Not usually." From very young ages, children can discriminate between different environments and understand that different rules apply. Consider the 3-year-old who knows that Daddy is a pushover and Mommy is stricter. The child usually knows that Daddy is the one to ask about getting ice cream or a new toy. This demonstrates that children learn early that different situations have different rules or conditions. Another illustration of this point is that parents of children who are often rude and out of control at home often hear from other parents that their children were cooperative and helpful while visiting the other parents' homes.

This is true of play sessions as well. In CCPT, the therapist reinforces the idea that the sessions are different from daily life as part of the structuring statement, in the phrase "This is a very special room" or "This is a very special playtime." Because children are able to express many things during play sessions that are not permitted in daily life, it seems that their needs are met better and that they actually reduce the maladaptive ways they have tried to meet their needs. Rather than exacerbating behavioral problems, it seems that CCPT sessions reduce or eliminate them. As children feel understood and their needs are met more fully, they no longer need to use inappropriate behaviors to express themselves. This outcome is enhanced when therapists help parents become better at hearing and reacting to their children's needs as well.

At times, however, it is possible that children may attempt play session behaviors in real life where such behaviors are not appropriate. In these cases, therapists usually inform parents that they should set limits on these behaviors as usual, or help them improve their limit-setting approach to address the behaviors. It would not be unusual for a limit-testing child to use the looser play session rules to try to get his or her own way: "But Cindy lets me do it in *her* playroom!" Therapists can give parents the language to counteract this: "Well, that's when you're having your special playtimes with Cindy. This is the rest of your life, and you may not do that now." This response is usually sufficient to help contain the behavior in question. It is useful for therapists to invite parents to report any "spillover effects," so that they can discuss ways to handle these rare occurrences.

Therapist Discomfort

As noted at several points in this chapter, there are times when children's behavior causes discomfort for therapists, either physically or psychologically. Sometimes therapists must weigh children's requests against their own discomfort, deciding whether or not they should learn to "stretch" themselves to be more accepting of a particular behavior. At other times, a limit is clearly needed, and this applies to situations in which therapists cannot overcome their own feelings of discomfort.

Generally such variations to the CCPT process are classified under the use of "personal limits," or those limitations imposed by a therapist due to his or her own special circumstances. For example, one play therapist set a personal limit about jumping rope, because she had had extensive knee surgery, and her knee could not take the pounding that comes with jumping rope. However, she did let the children know that she could skip rope gently, as this did not hurt her knee. Thus she was still able to follow the children's lead and direction, with a slight limitation.

Another example involves a therapist who had sustained a traumatic face injury in a car accident. He still flinched and experienced slight posttraumatic reactions when objects came through the air toward his face. He found it difficult to maintain an accepting stance when children unexpectedly or suddenly threw or tossed balls or other typically safe toys toward him. He was unable to convey full acceptance, as his flinching and startle reflex were very strong. In this case, he set a personal limit: "One of the rules in the special playtime is that you must first tell me before throwing that ball toward me."

This chapter has outlined some of the common questions and difficulties in conducting CCPT. When therapists encounter unclear situations, these are excellent times to seek supervision or case consultation. Perhaps one of the best ways of developing high-level skill at conducting CCPT is an ongoing supervision process with a qualified and experienced CCPT therapist.

CHAPTER 11

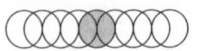

Touch in Child-Centered
Play Therapy

Touch is an essential part of all human existence. In its purest form, touch is a powerful form of communication and social bonding. Through touch, human beings and other animals can communicate either love and care or displeasure and disapproval. Children rely on touch from loving and safe caregivers to help them grow and develop. There have been horrific reports of badly neglected infants and children left alone in a form of "solitary confinement," never held or touched by another human being. The results of this neglect are significant developmental delays and sometimes even death. Research has shown that touch is essential for strengthening the parent–child attachment bond, promoting physiological development, and minimizing the effects of stress on infants (Jernberg & Booth, 1999).

Most people recognize that it feels good when a trusted friend or family member physically touches them in a warm and sincere way. Children gravitate to adults for the physical comfort of touch when they are upset, injured, or fearful. Every adult who has had experiences with children knows the power of "kissing a boo-boo" to make it better. Infants and children touch their own bodies to explore themselves and learn where they end and the rest of the world begins. Touch enables children to develop a sense of self, mastery of self and environment, and self-esteem. When touch is used appropriately, children flourish. When touch is used inappropriately, it can interfere with development or cause harm that can lead to lifelong problems for a child. It is important for all child therapists, including those using CCPT, to understand the significance of touch in therapy. Such understanding enables therapists to use touch appropriately, thereby meeting children's needs and enhancing the therapeutic process.

The Role of Touch in CCPT

Although touch can play a highly important role in the CCPT process, play therapists need to evaluate their reasons for using or not using touch. People have differing levels of comfort with touch, and it is important for play therapists to be aware of their own comfort levels. A therapist uncomfortable with any type of touch may experience some difficulties when using CCPT, and these issues need to be explored with a well-trained supervisor. CCPT therapists also need to ensure that their attitudes about and use of touch in play therapy are in the service of each individual child's needs, are in the child's best interests, and are consistent with the child's therapeutic goals. In other words, the use of touch involves a balance among several factors: respect for/understanding of a child's needs for touch, the play therapist's own comfort levels, and the rationale for any type of touch within the CCPT process.

Touch can become part of CCPT in many different ways and contexts. The type of touch that is permissible is determined by the play therapist, although the child is generally the one who initiates touch in CCPT. One exception to this rule is when a child is refusing to end a play session. In such cases, the CCPT therapist must act, often utilizing touch, to bring the session to an end. For example, Toby was a 5-year-old boy who had difficulty with transitions and was a masterful limit tester. He was the type of child for whom all therapists should be prepared— one likely to make quite a fuss when the time was up and he had to leave the special room.

As described in Chapter 5 of this book, it is always wise to start with the least intrusive means of ending the session. That is, the play therapist stands up and says it's time to go. In Toby's case, he continued to play at the table, ignoring the play therapist's announcement and nonverbal signals that the session was over. When he disregarded the play therapist's usual ending cues, the therapist approached Toby, touched him on the shoulder, and said, "It's hard to end the session when you are having such a good time. Our time is up, so we have to go." Toby quickly grabbed a toy in each hand and stated, "I'm not leaving unless I can take these with me." The play therapist acknowledged, "It's really hard for you to leave, so you want to take those toys with you. Remember the rule is that you can't take any toys from the playroom," and the therapist gently pried each toy out of Toby's hand. At that point, Toby grabbed onto the leg of the child-sized table with both hands and said he wouldn't leave. The play therapist had no choice but to carefully pry his little hands off the table leg and scoop him up in her arms, carrying Toby kicking and screaming out of the playroom. Throughout this time, the play therapist was acknowledging, "You hate when it is time to end. You're angry that you can't stay and play longer. It is really upsetting when you can't get what you want." By the time the therapist went through the playroom door carrying Toby, he was much calmer and realized that he had no choice but to accept the ending limit. This sequence is a completely acceptable use of touch to enforce the ending limit. Such issues with transitions and limit testing are best handled therapeutically by the consistent use of appropriate structure and enforcement of consequences when the child does not comply.

Because some touching is necessary to enforce consequences, all child therapists, including play therapists, should obtain training in appropriate methods for touching or lightly restraining children. This ensures that the least intrusive methods are used, and that neither a child nor a therapist is injured.

In some ways, physically removing a recalcitrant child from the special room can be easier to manage than other forms of touch. There are many times children want to be touched, and at some of these times, a child's desire for touch may be inappropriate. Examples are probably the best way to help novice play therapists learn about when to use touch. For example, if a child wants to suck on a baby bottle while being held by the therapist "like a baby," there is no reason not to follow the child's lead and fulfill the request (provided, of course, that the therapist can provide a clean baby bottle for this purpose). If the child tries to touch the play therapist's breast as he or she cuddles and sucks on the bottle, a limit needs to be set restricting the child from touching the therapist in that way. The therapist might say to the child, "You really enjoy being held while you suck on the bottle. Remember there are some rules. One rule is that you cannot touch my breasts while we cuddle. But you can do almost anything else."

It should be noted that some touching behavior that may be acceptable between a parent and a child in FT may not be appropriate between a CCPT therapist and a child. One example is of a 3-year-old girl named Myra, who had been sexually abused by her father. One of Myra's presenting symptoms was that she often had stomachaches stemming from the abuse. During the play therapy session with her mother, Myra often wanted her mother to hold her like a baby and rub her belly because it hurt. Her mother followed Myra's lead and did as Myra asked. The belly rubbing by her mother served to decrease Myra's anxiety, allowing Myra to feel sufficiently comforted to resume playing. Although Myra never made a similar request of the play therapist, this would have been a situation where the therapist would exercise caution. Because of Myra's strong attachment to her mother, Myra was able to interpret the belly rubbing as nurturing and supportive. This would have been far less likely with the play therapist, who played adjunctively with Myra to build trust and relationship so that Myra could eventually feel safe enough to reveal the story of her abuse to the therapist. Because of Myra's sexual abuse history, an individual CCPT therapist would be likely to experience some discomfort with the intimacy of this kind of contact. The play therapist would want to limit this type of touch, simply because of the level of intimacy and the possibility that this could trigger Myra to experience a reenactment of the abuse by her father.

Other positive forms of touch include a child's spontaneously (1) hugging the play therapist, (2) leaning against the play therapist while completing some artwork, (3) putting a hand up for a high-five after an accomplishment, or (4) taking the play therapist's hand to enter or exit the playroom. The therapist should respond empathically to all of these touch interactions, so that the child experiences the physical closeness with comfort, while the play therapist's acceptance signals that this type of touch is permissible. For example, the therapist might say, "You like to hold hands with me while we go out."

It is important to remember that any touch may be uncomfortable for some children—as it was for Damian, a 10-year-old boy diagnosed with mild Asperger syndrome, tactile defensiveness, and limit-testing tendencies. At the end of one session, Damian continued to play after being told the session was over for that day. When he did not leave the room, the play therapist touched him on the shoulder to indicate that it was time to go. Damian responded, "Don't touch me. You know I don't like to be touched." The play therapist acknowledged this, but reiterated that the session was over and they had to leave. Once they were out of the playroom, the therapist used this moment therapeutically by acknowledging to Damian his discomfort with being touched, and stating that she would remember not to touch him if he would remember to leave just as soon as it was announced that time was up. Damian agreed, and a brief conversation ensued in which Damian made the connection that people such as teachers and peers did things such as using touch that made him uncomfortable when he did not comply with a request made of him. Ultimately, Damian agreed that if he wanted people to respect his personal boundaries, he needed to learn to respect the boundaries of others.

Risks of Touch in CCPT

Play therapists need to recognize that touch has become a highly sensitive topic today. With widespread Internet access, people have more access to children than ever. Along with such access comes the potential for danger. Television programs such as "To Catch a Predator" on NBC's *Dateline* have served to heighten parents' awareness and fears that their children may be potential victims. Play therapists must be aware that they can be suspected of child abuse if parents perceive the play therapist's actions in play therapy or helping a child in the bathroom as inappropriate touch. Living in a highly litigious society requires that we pay close attention to our use of touch and keep parents informed of our policies regarding touch. Unfortunately, even well-meaning play therapists can become victims of aggressive parents who see financial opportunity in the form of malpractice litigation.

An experience one of us had years ago serves as an example of this. Using FT, the therapist met with a single mother who had four children ranging in age from 6 to 11. The oldest child was confined to a wheelchair because of a degenerative condition. At the first and second sessions, the mother talked at great length about how her disabled son required a great deal of help with toileting. The mother appeared to be overwhelmed with this son's care. When pressed, she did acknowledge that the two middle children were capable of helping their older brother in the bathroom. During the third session, the mother was conducting her first FT play session with the youngest child when the 10-year-old daughter, Alicia, knocked on the door of the observation room. When the therapist answered the door, Alicia stated that her brother had to go to the bathroom and needed the therapist's help. Oddly, when the therapist went out to the waiting room, all three children insisted that she be the one to help him go to the toilet. The therapist gently explained that she understood he needed help, but that she needed to watch their mother's play session. The therapist further explained that their mother had told her that they were capable of helping him, and she returned to her observation. At the end of the mother's play sessions, the therapist gave her feedback; she made sure to mention the request for help with the eldest son in the bathroom and how she had handled it. Although the mother rescheduled for the following week, she did not appear for the next session, never called to cancel, and never returned the therapist's phone calls to her. It was then that the therapist realized that the mother had probably tried to set her up, and (with the assistance of her children) had put the therapist in a potentially risky situation. In this case, the therapist's intuition, most likely guided by her perceptions that the children's behaviors were odd, helped her avoid falling victim to a potential legal scam.

This story is not intended to scare play therapists away from the use of touch, but rather to make sure that they carefully analyze potential risks. *Touch is only appropriate when it is driven solely by the needs of the child; is consistent with the treatment goals; and does not violate any ethical, moral, or professional standards.*

Any type of sexual contact or erotic touch is clearly off limits in the context of CCPT or any child therapy. CCPT therapists also need to be mindful of their own reactions and refrain from touch in situations where they may feel sexually aroused by a child's play, uncomfortable with the type of touch a child is seeking, or feeling angry toward a child. It is important as well to exercise caution in situations where the child may misconstrue the touch as sexual, aggressive, or punitive.

One example of the need for mindfulness regarding touch occurred when Lance, a 16-year-old boy with severe developmental delays, was seen in CCPT. The therapist described how she was sitting in a child-sized chair with her legs crossed when her high-heeled shoe inadvertently slipped off her foot. Because of her full engagement in the process of the child's play, the play therapist noted that Lance became aroused and started to lightly touch his penis over his clothes. She immediately acknowledged to Lance that it felt good when he touched himself, but she added a limit on this behavior in the context of the special room. Lance responded that he wanted her to take off her shoe so he could touch her foot, which was clearly the trigger for Lance's erotic behavior. Again, the play therapist accepted Lance's feelings, but limited the behavior; this allowed Lance to resume his normal play. At the end of the session, the play therapist informed Lance's mother of what had occurred. Though embarrassed, the mother admitted that her son had a foot fetish, and that she was deeply concerned about it. This opened the door for the therapist to help the mother learn how to set appropriate limits on this behavior.

Special Considerations for Traumatized Children

The use of touch with physically and/or sexually abused children in CCPT deserves special consideration. The use of touch with traumatized children must be approached with thoughtfulness and care. A child's need for touch in appropriate ways can help the child resolve the symptoms of trauma and reconfigure any maladaptive coping strategies the child may have developed as a result of the abuse. Once touch has been used to hurt a child, that child is often confused about how to distinguish between good (appropriate) and bad (inappropriate) touch.

One example involved a 6-year-old boy named Corey who had been sodomized by his father. The mother reported that Corey had become very clingy and seemed to crave physical closeness. Although she had done some reading with him on "good" touch versus "bad" touch, Corey would occasionally touch her inappropriately. The mother worked with the therapist to learn how to set appropriate limits on "bad" touch, while helping Corey learn the type of touch acceptable to her so that his needs for touch could be met. During this confusing period, Corey's play sessions focused on touch. For example, he often tentatively leaned against the play therapist or asked if he could lay his head on her lap. The play therapist actively acknowledged his feelings, using statements such as "You're not sure if it's okay to lean against me," or "You're wondering if it's okay to lay your head on my lap." When Corey answered "Yes" to these empathic responses, the play therapist reminded him, "You can do almost anything you want in the special room. If there's something you can't do, I will tell you." This simple structure gave Corey a sense of safety that he had lost during the abuse, when boundaries were blurred by his father's inappropriateness.

It is important to remember that in CCPT touch is always child-driven, though the play therapist is responsible for ensuring that the type of touch is appropriate and that clear limits are set regarding inappropriate touch. A training group of child therapists who specialized in working with sexually abused children raised several good questions about touch and how to handle various situations with this traumatized population. The therapists stated that many of their child clients used touch inappropriately or asked them to touch the children in inappropriate ways. They also asked about the appropriateness of having a child reenact a sexual act, such as touching a doll's genital areas. In CCPT, there is a distinction between a child's fantasy play and real-life reenactments. A child's fantasy play is generally allowed, just as long as the fantasy play does not evolve into behaviors that would call for a limit. For example, it would be okay for the child to undress a doll and even touch the doll's private areas. The play therapist would actively respond by stating, "You're taking off the doll's clothes to see it naked. You're curious about that. You want to touch the doll's penis to see what that's like." Often, too, children act out behaviors through fantasy play that were part of their sexual abuse because they want to see the play therapist's reaction. If that appears to be the case, the play therapist should respond, "You're wondering what I think about you touching the doll's penis." If pressed by the child to answer, the therapist can say, "You can do almost anything you'd like in the special room, and I'll let you know if there's something you can't do." On the other hand, if a child sits on the bop bag and begins moving back and forth as if masturbating, the therapist sets a limit: "You like the way that feels, but one of the things you may not do is rub yourself on the bop bag." If a boy wants to take his own pants down to rub his penis against the doll, a limit is also stated, because it would be inappropriate for the child to expose his genitals during the play session. Similarly, it would not be appropriate for the child to expect the play therapist to expose his or her genitals, nor should there ever be any sexual contact between the child and the play therapist. Also, the play therapist does not engage in fantasy play where the therapist would physically reenact sexual behaviors, as this would send a very confusing message to the child about the appropriateness of such adult behavior. If the child asks the therapist to hold him or her around the waist very tightly and not to let go, the therapist declines this role as well. If the child is confused as to why he or she is allowed to participate in sexual fantasy play, but the play therapist will not cooperate with this request, the confusion needs to be acknowledged. The play therapist can state, "I don't feel comfortable doing that, because it's not okay for grownups to hurt children that way."

Because this is a confusing area for many therapists, an example with several levels of behavior is used below to illustrate how CCPT therapists handle children's sexualized play. The example differentiates between the use of limits for inappropriate behavior and empathic listening for the child's therapeutic work—in this case, a reenactment of sexual abuse.

Johnny asked his therapist if she wanted to see what was under his pants, and without waiting for an answer, he began to remove his pants. The therapist set a limit: "Johnny, in the special playroom, you will always keep your clothes on and I will always keep my clothes on, so that our private parts are covered. I will never ask to see or touch your private parts, and I will not show you my private parts. This is a place where everyone keeps their clothes on to stay safe and comfortable." Then Johnny took two dolls and undressed them. The therapist reflected, "You're taking off their clothes, and now they're naked." Johnny then said that one doll didn't like to be naked, but the other doll made her do it. The therapist said, "Oh. She is uncomfortable. This naked thing wasn't her idea. She didn't feel like she had a choice." Johnny replied, "No. The big girl would hurt her if she said no." The therapist continued reflecting: "It sounds like she is really scared, and there was no one there to help. She wishes she could get out of there." Johnny then placed the perpetrator doll on top of the smaller doll and moved them up and down. The therapist said, "That big girl is moving up and down on the little girl. She must be really confused and scared."

In this case, the therapist set a limit on real-time behaviors that were inappropriate, but she accepted and empathically listened to the imaginary play, being careful to stay within the metaphor Johnny created. It is important for a therapist to remember that this type of play represents the child's work. The child is processing the abuse. The therapist must be reflective rather than reactive. When a therapist shows discomfort or limits the child's imaginary play, this runs the risk of increasing the child's shame, guilt, anxiety, and confusion associated with the abuse. In essence, stopping such play just as the child is symbolically reenacting the trauma amounts to colluding with the secrecy of abuse. Children often cannot talk about these experiences, as it is too threatening to do so; CCPT may offer the one opportunity they have to communicate and work through their feelings of fear, helplessness, anger, and confusion. Supervision with a CCPT therapist who has experience in treating abused children can help therapists discuss their own reactivity, so they are in a better position to be accepting and helpful to these children.

Informing Parents and Documenting Touch in CCPT

As stated earlier, touch has become a highly sensitive topic in our society. Therefore, before therapy begins, it is wise to inform parents that some types of touch may occur during CCPT; that the use of touch is driven by the needs of the child; and that any sexual or erotic touch is forbidden between the child and play therapist. It is equally important to inform parents that the therapist may need to use touch (i.e., guiding a child by the hand or carrying a child out of the room, to enforce the ending boundary). Furthermore, the play therapist needs to assure the parents that every incident of touch will be explained to the parents after the session, including how the touch was initiated and addressed, and the subsequent consequence or reaction of the child. After any incident of touch during the CCPT session, the incident and its explanation to parents should be clearly documented in the play therapist's notes. For their own protection, play therapists may want to consider devising a document of informed consent that includes a section on physical contact between the child and play therapist, and have parents sign this written release form.

When in doubt about how to handle issues of touch, supervision or case consultation with a Registered Play Therapist-Supervisor is the best course of action. The issue of touch is complex, as a CCPT therapist must consider not only the needs of the child, but also his or her own history, needs, feelings, thoughts, and motivations. It is important to remember that therapists' understanding of themselves as individuals serves to clarify who they are as CCPT therapists and enable them to make appropriate decisions regarding the use of touch in CCPT.

The Association for Play Therapy (*www.a4pt.org*) updates a "Paper on Touch: Clinical, Professional, and Ethical Issues" approximately every 3 years. Available as a .pdf on the website, it covers all the relevant issues regarding touch, and provides an excellent reference list for therapists interested in other resources on the topic of touch.

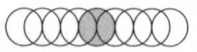

CHAPTER 12

Cultural and Systemic Considerations in the Practice of Child-Centered Play Therapy

Because interest in play therapy has grown substantially throughout the world, and because the United States and other countries have become much more culturally diverse in recent years, it is important for therapists to be aware of cultural issues that might affect their CCPT work with children and families. Similarly, child and family therapists' work is often embedded within or relevant to other systems, such as schools, communities, funding streams, or government services. Play therapists often face challenges that relate to these other services or environments in which children are involved. For example, many therapists complain that they feel pressured to resolve even entrenched child problems very quickly. Sometimes the coordination of CCPT and other child therapy efforts with other service delivery systems, such as child protective services or residential programs, becomes confused by lack of communication. This chapter addresses the cultural relevance of CCPT, as well as some of the common systemic challenges to the use of CCPT and possible means of overcoming them.

Cultural Relevance

All three of us authors and many of our play therapy colleagues have trained and worked with culturally diverse groups in the United States and abroad. Increasingly, play therapy associations and other professional groups are arising in many countries with the aim of training therapists and supporting the practice of play therapy. Even within the United States, children from many different cultural backgrounds need treatment, and play therapists must be culturally aware and sensitive so that their interventions "fit" with each child's family and cultural environments.

For the purposes of this discussion, "culture" refers to a family's history; racial identity and ethnic heritage; and customs, beliefs, and practices. It is important to remember that even within specific racial or ethnic groups, there is tremendous variation, and generalizations must be avoided. Each individual and each family need to be considered for their own unique character and customs. In fact, it is useful to remember that all families have their own unique cultural beliefs and practices, which are embedded within the broader culture and society in which they live and work. Therapists must be respectful, sensitive, and accepting of the individuality and diversity of each child, parent, and family with whom they work. The empathy that is so important to CCPT and FT is critical for developing collaborative relationships and showing understanding for all families.

People's cultural backgrounds affect the ways they see things and do things. Therapy usually involves making some changes to family dynamics, and perhaps the most culturally sensitive interventions are those in which parents are engaged as partners in the process. In this way, therapists listen carefully to their input and discuss the "fit" of interventions with the parents' worldviews. A genuine partnership with parents is much more likely to yield culturally relevant and appropriate interventions. Gil and Drewes (2005) have explored this fascinating and vital arena in their book *Cultural Issues in Play Therapy*, and other excellent resources are available as well (e.g., Ellis & Carlson, 2009). A few points relevant to CCPT and FT are included below.

All children play if given the opportunity. Play is universal and appears to serve key developmental purposes for children everywhere. CCPT seems particularly well suited to children from various cultural backgrounds because of its nondirective nature. In a playroom stocked with a wide range of toys, children are free to play as they choose.

Because children are embedded in their culture, their play reflects their perceptions of that cultural environment. Well-trained therapists appreciate this uniqueness, and they respond in ways that show acceptance of each child's individuality. An important goal is for children to accept themselves, and this includes acceptance of their own racial or ethnic identity.

For example, a 7-year-old African American boy, Sam, consistently set aside a set of dark-skinned puppets and selected light-skinned ones to play with during his early FT play sessions with his African American parents. His parents used their empathy skills to be accepting of his choices, but they shared their concerns with the therapist. Sam's behavior seemed so deliberate that it appeared he was rejecting the puppets whose skin color was similar to his own. The therapist empathically listened to the parents and urged them to trust that the FT process would probably provide more clues about his feelings over time. In the fourth session of this nature, Sam began to play with one of the dark-skinned puppets. Two of the lighter-skinned puppets began to make fun of the dark-skinned one. His mother reflected the scene really well: "Those girls are making fun of his dark skin. They are teasing him. . . . He is very hurt. Now he is calling them names. He's angry and sad about all this." In the postsession discussion, the therapist and parents hypothesized that problems like the ones Sam had enacted might be happening at school. Together they developed a plan for the parents to discuss this possibility with the teacher and school counselor. The therapist also encouraged the parents to consider ways they could do some activities together as a family that might help their son begin to see his race in a more positive light. Most important, perhaps, was the way in which Sam began to resolve his own struggle. In subsequent play sessions, he began to empower the dark-skinned character more and more, and it appeared that he was working out some of his feelings that stemmed from the teasing.

One area where cultural factors often play a role is in the interpretation of a child's play. As noted in the discussion of play themes in Chapter 6, it is critical to make only tentative interpretations, with full consideration of the context in which the child lives. Children play within their cultural context, and parents are in a good position to discuss this with therapists. Parents have knowledge and insight about possible meanings of children's play, so when they are engaged regularly during CCPT or fully in FT, they often can shed light on what meanings the play might have for the child. The parents know the unique cultural features of their family. For example, during a grandparent–child play session in FT, a 4-year-old boy became fascinated with the rubber chicken and a small basket of eggs. He played intently with them for several minutes, eventually asking his grandmother several times, "Do these eggs really crack?" The child had many attachment issues because of sporadic parenting by his mentally ill mother. The grandmother, who took care of the child regularly, was able to offer a possible interpretation of this egg play that a therapist might never have considered. The grandmother commented, "Whenever he comes to visit me, I usually like to bake something nice for him. I give him little jobs to help with the baking, and one of them is cracking the eggs." With this information about the family context (the egg-cracking and baking routine), the therapist and grandmother hypothesized that his egg play and questions were possibly related to his role in the family and how seriously he took his egg-cracking job. The grandmother was also pleased that her nurturance efforts meant so much to him. Without the family context, known only to the grandmother, the therapist could have remained in the dark about the most likely meaning of this play.

Of utmost importance, however, is the creation of an open, genuine, and collaborative relationship with parents. Therapists must adopt an attitude of humility. They do not "know it all," nor should they. All clients have much important information to share, and when therapists empathize and encourage transcultural dialogue with parents, their work is enriched—made more relevant by their acknowledgment of individual and family identity, culture, and uniqueness.

Misunderstanding of CCPT by Other Professionals

Other mental health or medical professionals are not always aware of CCPT or how it works, and even play therapists who have not had substantial training in the method can develop misunderstandings about it. We have heard many claims about CCPT that reflect the speakers' opinions but that are not well grounded in theory or research. Some have claimed that CCPT is not appropriate for children with trauma or attachment issues. Others seem to believe that CCPT provides a "free-for-all" for children, without setting boundaries or limits on their destructive behaviors. Still others have stated that CCPT is no longer viable in an age of short-term therapy. Such claims generally reveal a lack of understanding of high-quality CCPT practice. When practitioners hear such claims, they should question them, evaluate the source documents that are referenced, and/or discuss them with experienced and qualified CCPT supervisors. Upon closer examination, we have found that some claims simply do not stand up, for one or more of these reasons: Insufficient research is cited; the research that is cited uses dubious methodology; the description provided of CCPT bears scant similarity to CCPT as it is properly defined and practiced; or those providing the therapy in the research, those presenting the research, or both have not had significant training in CCPT.

Therefore, child practitioners need to consider all claims about CCPT (positive or negative) with a bit of skepticism, followed by a firsthand examination of any evidence provided—including whether or not CCPT was actually used, the extent of training and qualification of the study's therapists, the research design employed, and the accuracy of the conclusions. Chapter 13 provides further guidance in evaluating research, as well as a summary of the empirical research to date on CCPT or FT. Ultimately, CCPT therapists who obtain high-quality training and supervised practice are in a better position to judge the impact of the approach for themselves.

Pressures for Quick Results

CCPT therapists sometimes feel pressured by referral sources, parents, or insurance companies to achieve fast outcomes. It can be easy to succumb to such pressures, either by trying to hurry the therapy along or by feeling inadequate because others' expectations cannot be met. Understanding the sources of the "quick-fix" pressure helps therapists to handle this situation better and to remain true to the best interests of their child clients.

Some pressure for fast results is probably driven by financial motives. Some insurance companies seem to be set up to make more profits by approving fewer services or sessions; government funding provides limited resources to spread over many families in need; and some bureaucracies seem to consume more funding than they give out. In these cases, the funding for CCPT can be insufficient, or therapists must frequently justify their need for more sessions. Here it is helpful to educate the gatekeepers and to express some of the advantages of CCPT in financial terms.

For example, one insurance company began *recommending* FT after it saw the typical outcomes. This company also liked the psychoeducational nature of FT and its prior studies of long-term effectiveness. A key individual in this company was introduced to FT by a therapist, and this gatekeeper subsequently educated other decision makers within the company. Sometimes insurance companies have gradually learned about CCPT and other play therapy approaches when their own employees have benefited from such services.

Similarly, one play therapist in a community mental health center educated the county and state program evaluators about how CCPT and FT address the root causes of many child problems. She also showed them how these approaches reduced the "revolving-door" phenomenon, in which clients (1) came to the center in crisis, (2) were given short-term "fixes" that they only partially implemented at home, (3) dropped out of therapy prematurely because the crisis passed and/or the treatment was not helping, and (4) showed up again a few months later with a new crisis. The developmentally more appropriate CCPT (and other forms of play therapy coupled with parent skills training, as discussed in Chapter 2 and 8 of this volume) led to better outcomes for many families, which in turn improved family involvement and follow-through with treatment. FT in particular yielded positive results that the officials had not seen before. Eventually the program evaluators became enthusiastic about play therapy approaches that required additional resources in the short run but fewer in the long run.

When parents and school personnel express the need for a "quick fix," this is likely to stem from frustration with and concern for a child's behavior. Sometimes they have waited until they are quite desperate to make the referral for therapy. Their pressure for fast results is more likely to be an expression of their helplessness, because all they have tried has failed.

In this situation, the CCPT therapist must first listen empathically to their concerns and feelings. A thorough understanding of parents' and/or teachers' frustrations can assist the therapist in making more helpful responses. For example, the therapist might suggest a school observation and consultation to help teachers manage the child's disruptiveness. Only when parents or teachers feel truly "heard" will they be able to hear the therapist's realistic appraisal of the situation. The therapist can then educate them about the situation and guide them toward positive actions, thereby restoring hope.

A therapist named Cassie began CCPT with a 6-year-old, Larry, who had frequent tantrums in his first-grade classroom after his father died suddenly from a heart attack. The mother was depressed, and FT was contraindicated because of her extremely low energy levels. After three CCPT sessions, Larry's mother told Cassie that the CCPT was "not working" and that Larry's teacher had threatened to suspend him if he could not control his outbursts. Cassie suspected that his mother felt inadequate, especially when the school seemed to be expecting change quickly. Cassie listened in an accepting and empathic way to the mother: "You really feel bad to hear this from the school. You were hoping we could get these tantrums stopped right away. . . . Might it be helpful for me to talk directly with Larry's teacher and school counselors? Perhaps I could talk about what we're doing here and how you've been cooperating—and maybe we could even come up with some things that might help the teacher in the meantime."

Once the proper releases were signed, Cassie spoke with the teacher. Again, she listened carefully and empathically to the teacher's frustration and exasperation. After the teacher had vented and calmed down, Cassie explained how CCPT works and what to expect in terms of time frames for change; she then offered to consult with the school for some shorter-term remedies. A 45-minute meeting with Cassie, the mother, the teacher, and the school counselor led to an interim plan that satisfied everyone. One week of behavioral charts showed the times and circumstances most likely to result in tantrums. The teacher implemented a simple reinforcement plan, and the counselor began to see Larry for in-school support. This satisfied the teacher, removed pressure from the mother, and gave the CCPT time to work. Larry used his CCPT sessions fully, often playing out imaginary father–son football games as well as burial scenes in the sandtray. By his 12th session, his teacher reported that the tantrums were greatly reduced.

CCPT is not necessarily long-term therapy. For children to work through the process of exploring the playroom, aggressive play, regressive and other theme-related play, and mastery play, a minimum of 10 half-hour sessions is recommended. (The other half-hour of a typical therapy hour can be spent in working with parents or conducting other child or family interventions.) In their meta-analysis, Bratton et al. (2005) found that most nondirective play therapists averaged 22 sessions with their clients. Of course, some complex or deeply rooted problems take longer, but CCPT is not by definition a long-term approach.

CCPT with Children
in Foster or Protective Care

Children who have been placed in the foster care system have experienced maltreatment and attachment disruptions that affect their subsequent adjustment. They have many emotional and social needs. Sometimes the system designed to protect them is inadequately prepared to meet those needs, and cases of abuse within the system have even been reported (Bernstein, 2001). Funding can be inadequate for full rehabilitation; staff members may have heavy caseloads; and staff training programs may not provide a solid foundation on the impact of trauma and attachment disruption on children. Without this foundation, it is common for caseworkers, foster parents, and residential program staff to interpret children's disruptive behaviors too simplistically as "bad," without a full understanding of the social and emotional components underlying those behaviors. This misinterpretation of trauma-reactive behaviors can lead to less-than-optimal decisions for the children, and when desired results are not achieved, frustration levels can increase for all involved.

Providing mental health treatment of any type to children in the foster/protective care system can be challenging, not only because many of these children present trauma-reactive problems, but also because of systemic inadequacies such as those described above. Furthermore, in many places, there is a history of tension between mental health care providers and protective services agencies. These tensions probably arise from the inherent difficulty of the work, inadequate funding, and a lack of understanding of the respective agencies' differing goals and foci. In other words, it is often a systemic problem that becomes more personalized when service providers share responsibility for a child who is difficult to manage. For a variety of reasons, communication and coordination can be quite poor, and many child therapists complain that they are not consulted before important decisions about children's lives and placements are made. This can result in poor or even disastrous results for a child, as the following case example illustrates.

Nick was in foster care after being abandoned by his father and physically abused by his mother's paramours. At age 6, he had many signs of trauma and attachment disruption, including oppositional and aggressive behaviors. He engaged quickly and worked very well in CCPT. He used the play sessions to work through his historic traumatic experiences, and he invited the therapist to join his play. In the imaginary roles, he offered to protect her from the many dangers surrounding them, and he gained mastery over his fears by enacting powerful, protective roles. An extended course of CCPT lasting over a year resulted in gains noticed by both his foster mother and the child protective services agency that managed his case.

After a period of considerable progress, his foster mother reported increased aggression and destructive behaviors at home. Nick eventually disclosed to the therapist that a teenage relative of his foster mother had come to live with them. This boy had sexually assaulted him, and Nick then disclosed prior sexual abuse in a previous foster placement. Nick was very attached to his foster mother, who had been planning to adopt him. They shared an ethnic heritage, and this allowed Nick to continue to hear his native language spoken, eat familiar foods, and feel comfortable with extended family rituals and events. After the abuse was disclosed, the therapist reported it as mandated; the decision was made to place Nick in another home, primarily because the perpetrator was continuing to reside at the home.

The foster mother was so distraught about losing Nick, however, that she could not bring herself to tell him that he would be leaving her. The therapist was unaware of this. Furthermore, with the full knowledge of the foster care agency, arrangements had been made for Nick to be dropped off at his next therapy appointment with a bag of his belongings, whereupon he would meet his new foster mother and go home with her. Neither Nick nor the therapist knew any of this. After dropping him off, the foster mother left without saying good-bye.

Nick was very hurt, scared, and confused by this course of events. When the new foster mother arrived, Nick was inconsolable, ran out of the office, and had to be located. The therapist was also distressed that she had not been informed of this, so that she could have facilitated the process. She notified the agency of her grave concern about the potential damaging impact of this lack of communication and coordination.

When Nick returned to therapy, he refused to go into the playroom where he had done so much work in the past year. He acted out in his new home and refused to enter the playroom for several weeks. Nick associated the playroom and the therapist with the traumatic separation from the foster mother with whom he had shared a strong attachment. The therapist had to create a new play area in a group meeting room to work with Nick, and it took nearly 4 months for her to reengage him fully in CCPT. Learning from this experience, the therapist requested meetings with the agency to discuss their relationship, the nature of therapy, and ways they could prevent such a situation from ever happening again.

As this case illustrates, CCPT practitioners often acquire valuable information about children that can be helpful for decision makers. For this reason, it is important that they be included as part of the decision-making team. When they feel excluded or dismissed by those making decisions, there are a couple of steps they can take. First, they can contact the appropriate case manager or agency liaison and ask to be included in all team meetings. They can offer to provide treatment summaries for use in decision making as well as in court reports. Sometimes this is sufficient to alert others of the need to include the therapists. Therapists must also find ways to strengthen and nurture their relationships with the relevant agencies.

Second, if significant tensions or negative attitudes exist between the foster/protective care agency and mental health care providers, it can be very beneficial to suggest some simple cross-training. Sometimes a 2-hour presentation about play therapy and the child therapist's role in the bigger picture can pave the way for much-improved collaboration and coordination. For example, one community mental health center offering play therapy services had a long history of bickering with the child protective services agency with which they shared many clients. Often this conflict surfaced when a particularly difficult case arose or when a client "fell through the cracks." The two organizations eventually held a series of cross-training sessions during which they shared information about their legal mandates, funding streams, challenges, and approaches to their work. Without a "hot case" facing them at the time, professionals from both organizations were able to gain a better appreciation of each other's work and limitations. A clearer understanding of play therapy led to increased referrals, improved communication, and fewer contentious moments between the two agencies. Eventually the child protective services agency asked play therapists from the mental health center to provide a play-based inservice day for their staff, in order to help them cope with their stressful jobs and to prevent vicarious traumatization!

This same educational approach can be applied to other organizations and individuals who are involved with children, families, and the decisions that affect their lives. Therapists who offer brief programs for domestic violence professionals, lawyers, judges, and guardians ad litem have reported benefits: more frequent inclusion in decision-making processes, as well as greater sensitivity to the psychosocial issues on the part of other professionals, including court-ordered recommendations for the appropriate therapies.

In general, when frustrations and faulty interactions occur between organizations working with very distressed children, it can signal a systems problem stemming from stresses inherent in the work or different mandates that seem at cross-purposes. In these cases, dialogues during less stressful times and other educational efforts are likely to pay off when more challenging situations arise, as they inevitably do.

Using CCPT in Conjunction with Directive Play Therapy Approaches

There are times when a play therapist who primarily uses CCPT sees the need to conduct some directive play therapy with certain children. Some settings, such as schools, are rather challenging for play therapy work because limited time and space are available (see the next section for more on conducting CCPT in such settings). Where many children require assistance in a limited time, therapists might opt for group play therapy or goal-focused cognitive-behavioral play therapy. Sometimes play therapists see the need for children to learn certain skills in order to optimize their coping. CCPT can be combined with directive play therapy, but because the interventions are based on different principles and assumptions, several issues must be considered.

When nondirective and directive play therapy approaches are combined, it is extremely important to ensure that a child knows the difference. The two forms of play therapy are combined only in sequence and never in the same moment. This prevents confusion for the child and keeps the "promises" made to the child intact. If therapists introduce CCPT with some form of the standard entry statement—"This is our special playtime. You may do almost anything you want, and if there's anything you may not do, I'll let you know"—they must honor the nondirective stance until they close that portion of the session with the time warnings and clear ending. It is never acceptable for the therapist to make suggestions in the middle of a CCPT session, as that represents a violation of the promise made in the entry statement.

In order to preserve the atmosphere of the "special room," it works best to reserve the playroom for CCPT and to use a separate office for more directive forms of play therapy. In a case where a play therapist has only one office for all types of child therapy, the therapist has to be a bit more creative about showing distinction between the CCPT and the more directive approaches being employed. One suggestion is that the toys for the CCPT be put away in a corner of the room or covered with a blanket, and thereby made off limits (except for the play therapist to extract toys that may be useful) during the more directive play therapy. Some therapists have divided their playrooms into a CCPT area and an "everything else" area where directive play therapy or art interventions can occur. The areas are divided by furniture or screens. One school counselor (C. Mader, personal communication, 1998) used a folding bookcase in her counseling room for this purpose. She placed toys for CCPT use on one side of the bookcase, and a small table and non-CCPT items on the other side. She used limit setting to keep children in whichever play area they were using at the moment.

Another way to avoid confusion (especially if the directive play therapy occurs immediately after the nondirective session) is to inform the child verbally of the distinction at the beginning of the session, and again when the therapy is changing from CCPT to the other activities planned. The therapist might start the session by saying, "For the first part today, *you* may select the toys and how you'd like to play with them; in the last part of today, I have some ideas of things we could do together." This would be followed by the usual CCPT entry statement. At the end of the CCPT session, the therapist would give the 5-minute and 1-minute warnings as usual, and then explain, "Now we're going to do something special that I've chosen that I think you'll like." Most children seem to adapt quite well to this arrangement. Even if the same room is used for everything, it is advisable to use a separate set of toys for each segment.

An example of directive play therapy used in conjunction with CCPT follows. Jonathan, age 10, was referred for treatment for acting out in school and oppositional defiance at home. Because the school planned to put him into a class for socially and emotionally disturbed children, the parents were desperate for quick answers to Jonathan's behavioral problems. In addition to CCPT once a week, Jonathan came to the office a second time during the same week to address some of his problematic behaviors directly. Role-playing social situations in which Jonathan typically became angry and reacted aggressively helped him learn interpersonal skills to express himself more appropriately. Bibliotherapy included an anger workbook with a cognitive-behavioral orientation; this helped Jonathan better understand how anger gets out of control. He also learned how to change his angry reactions by changing how he thought about things that made him angry. By changing his thoughts about trigger situations, Jonathan was able to reduce his angry feelings and make better decisions. The therapist also helped his parents improve their ability to establish appropriate limits, master consistency, and follow through with meaningful consequences. Although Jonathan's CCPT continued for many months, eight sessions including the directive approaches allowed him to remain in a regular classroom. These gains were consolidated by the CCPT sessions, wherein Jonathan was able to learn mastery of self, develop appropriate expression of feelings, and greatly improve his self-esteem.

When using nondirective and directive play therapy methods within a single session, therapists might wonder about the order in which to do this. In general, we believe that it is preferable to start with CCPT and end with more directive approaches. There are two main reasons for this. First, starting with CCPT gives children a chance to relax and permits freer expression of their own issues at the start of the session. It's the child-centered equivalent of the classic adult counseling lead-in: "Tell me how things have been going for you lately." Second, children typically leave therapy sessions to return to more structured environments, either at school or at home. Ending with the directive interventions provides a step toward greater structure, perhaps making that transition a bit easier.

Another question might arise about the respective length of time for these "split sessions" involving both CCPT and directive play therapy. We have found that a 30-minute CCPT session followed by a 10- or 15-minute directive play session is quite workable. If time is more restricted, a 20-minute CCPT session can be followed by a 10-minute directive segment. These suggestions are intended simply as guidelines.

Using CCPT in School, Hospital, or Home-Based Settings

CCPT is remarkably adaptable. It can be conducted in nearly any space where one can display a variety of toys. As we have noted in Chapter 4, one school counselor (C. Mader, personal communication, 1998) began holding her first CCPT sessions in a janitor's closet until there was more "buy-in" from teachers and administrators. When her sessions consistently resulted in better behavior in classrooms and at recess, teachers began telling her that they did not know what she was doing with the children, but that they wanted her to keep doing it. Over time, the school district invested in a van that served as a mobile play therapy vehicle. She drove it to the three schools where she provided counseling, and the children came out to the van for their play sessions, much as they might visit a Bookmobile to obtain library books.

In a children's crisis program where a dedicated playroom was not possible, two therapists (W. Caplin & K. Pernet, personal communication, 2004) adapted a large meeting room for FT play sessions. Using exercise mats in a rectangle on the floor to delineate the play space, they placed the toys on the mats and asked parents and children to play within the open area surrounded by the toy-covered mats. Similarly, one of us created a temporary CCPT space within a large group room by placing chairs in a circle, with the space enclosed by the chairs designated as the play area.

Although pediatric hospital settings often have a playroom for general use by inpatient children, it must remain open and available for everyone. Typically, these areas are not suitable for CCPT sessions. A mobile toy kit can be used in small consultation rooms or even in patient rooms. One therapist worked with chronically ill children on a pediatric floor of a medical center. When children were confined to their beds, she took toys into their rooms. A plastic storage box lined with rubber mats (to prevent the toys from rolling freely) and a box of miniature items were placed on a child's bed, and a portable dollhouse and play dishes were placed on the bedside tray table. The children, despite being very ill, played eagerly in the plastic box or with the toys on the tray table. The therapist sat beside the bed to conduct the CCPT sessions. Children could direct the therapist to bring various dress-up items (hats, sunglasses, and bandannas) and a mirror from a box placed on another chair nearby.

Home-based CCPT or FT is also possible, in which the entire therapy occurs within a family's home. This type of therapy can present unique challenges, however, as a therapist has little control over the home environment. Therapists typically use a portable toy kit and place items in a safe and private space. Bedrooms or other rooms where children play or spend a lot of time are not recommended. An effort is made to keep the therapy area separate from child-frequented areas, so that the distinction is clear between everyday play or other activities and the special therapeutic playtimes.

One challenge comes when the home environment is rather chaotic, with the television playing, other children running in and out, or neighbors visiting. A therapist conducting home-based sessions can help parents learn to manage the chaos by making suggestions or modeling behaviors that help calm the environment sufficiently to hold the play sessions. One therapist held home-based sessions in the family kitchen, but the other children kept interrupting from the dining room nearby. The therapist brought a small television and appropriate videos, which the other children watched in the dining room while he worked with the designated children one at a time. The therapist also helped the single mother adopt similar structuring methods when she needed to cook or handle other tasks without so many interruptions. Another challenge might be the unsuitability of the floor for play, perhaps because it is unclean or in poor repair. In this case, the therapist might conduct CCPT sessions on top of a wooden table, or incorporate the use of a washable vinyl table covering or sheet beneath the toys or seating areas.

Adaptability

There are usually ways to adapt CCPT and FT for most conditions. The *Casebook of Filial Therapy* (VanFleet & Guerney, 2003) contains numerous illustrations of clinical, cultural, and environmental adaptations therapists have made in order to conduct FT under a wide range of circumstances. When therapists confront difficulties in implementing these approaches, or when they encounter systemic problems or roadblocks, they should discuss the problems with other experienced CCPT therapists or supervisors. Furthermore, supervisors can provide the perspective, guidance, and support needed when challenges arise.

CCPT is a more complex intervention than many people realize. Supervisors can help therapists stay true to the principles; develop their CCPT skills; manage conflicts that arise; and build empathic, reciprocal, and effective relationships with families. These in turn help therapists serve children and families to the best of their abilities. Most CCPT professionals find their work exceptionally rewarding.

PART V

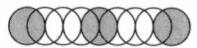

RESEARCH AND PROFESSIONAL ISSUES

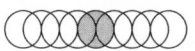

CHAPTER 13

Research on Child-Centered Play Therapy and Filial Therapy

Albert Einstein once said, "If we knew what we were doing, it wouldn't be called research, would it?" There is much about the practice of psychotherapy in general, and about play therapy in particular, that we do not know. Research is an ongoing process to determine outcomes and effectiveness, as well as which specific variables are most relevant to those outcomes under various circumstances. To serve children and families best, therapists must inform themselves of relevant research on the interventions that they use—and, when possible, conduct or participate in research that adds to the knowledge base.

An empirical base demonstrating the effectiveness of CCPT and FT has grown steadily through the years. This chapter briefly discusses the relative merits of different sources of clinical knowledge, and summarizes the principal research findings and resources to date.

Sources of Knowledge about Therapeutic Methods

Different forms of inquiry yield different types of information, all of which can be used to improve clinical practice. Reliance on a single source of information, whether it is one's own personal clinical experience or the most rigorously controlled research studies, fails to provide the fullest possible picture of the value of any intervention. In general, controlled research provides the strongest evidence of a therapeutic approach's efficacy, but other forms of data and information add details of use to clinicians as well.

The clinical experiences of thousands of child therapists provide information about the adaptability and applicability of a treatment method. On the one hand, therapeutic "fads" with little or no evidence rarely stand the test of time, fading in popularity if results are not forthcoming. On the other hand, treatments supported by rigorous research may not be adopted if they lack the flexibility and practicality needed in clinical work. Clinical evidence alone, however, is limited most significantly by therapist bias. Therapists want to feel that they are effective in their work, and it is likely that they view the results of their work through that lens, at least to some extent. Survey studies of therapists' use of CCPT provide information about how, where, and when they find it useful, but the results are likely to reflect self-report biases.

For example, if a survey showed that 80% of play therapists used CCPT with children with selective mutism, and 65% of those reported that children began whispering within eight sessions, clinicians might look more closely at CCPT as a possible treatment for their own cases of selective mutism. This survey, however, could not objectively reveal whether CCPT was truly effective with selective mutism; nor would it have predictive value for future cases of selective mutism.

Similarly, well-written individual case studies provide a level of detail that informs other clinicians of the subtleties of CCPT with a specific child or family situation, and the reactions of the individuals involved. Because some children and families share demographic and presenting problem features, professionals can see how the method might be applied in their own cases. Case studies can also be a source of new ideas worthy of further study, and they can demonstrate the flexible application of established methods.

Even so, there are many unique variables in each case situation, and one cannot generalize the outcomes from one case study to the next. On the other hand, as biologist and cognitive ethologist Marc Bekoff has noted, "The plural of case study is data." Multiple case studies using similar methods and yielding positive results should not be dismissed, for their combined data add to one's confidence that the method warrants consideration, despite the biases inherent in the case study approach.

Many surveys and case studies attest to the value of CCPT with a wide range of presenting problems in many different settings. The increased popularity of play therapy in recent years is attributable, at least in part, to clinicians' and families' sharing their enthusiasm for play therapy with others. This growing enthusiasm points professionals toward CCPT as a theoretically grounded, developmentally attuned therapeutic modality worthy of further consideration. Specific clinical case studies are not cited here, however, as their scientific value is limited and quite subjective in nature.

Quantitative research offers clinicians greater certainty about a treatment's objective effectiveness. Research designs controlling for many of the variables that potentially influence outcomes add confidence to the results. For example, results from a study performed with randomized assignment of sufficient numbers of clients to a specified treatment group and a waiting-list control group would be considered a reliable determination of the treatment's effectiveness. Quasi-experimental research designs using control or comparison groups offer considerably more certainty than those involving pretests and posttests of a single treatment group, although the latter are more informative than case reports that contain no measurements at all. Time series designs using multiple measurement points before, during, and after treatment would also control for many possible variables affecting outcomes. (A useful and classic resource on research design is Stanley & Campbell, 1973.) These more rigorous study designs are critical for establishing a treatment as "evidence-based" within the social science community, and they dramatically increase the attractiveness of an approach to program administrators and funders. A growing body of quantitative studies has clearly demonstrated the effectiveness of CCPT and FT, and these findings are summarized in the next section. By itself, however, this form of quantitative research does not give the whole picture.

Program evaluation studies are typically conducted in the "real world" under less-than-optimal conditions for research. Program evaluation research aims to determine the effectiveness of an operating program through the most controlled means possible, but practical and ethical challenges often reduce the ability to implement experimental designs. For example, one might wish to evaluate the usefulness of play therapy in a community mental health center. The center most likely has a system for determining how and when cases are assigned to clinicians, often based on urgency of need or length of time on a waiting list. In this case, the random assignment of children to treatment conditions could raise ethical issues, such as whether the study would require withholding or postponing play therapy for those who need it most. Often the use of a waiting-list control group strengthens program evaluation research, but it is not always possible. It is also difficult to use manualized protocols in such research, because of the unique and multiple needs of many families in clinical settings. The evaluation cannot deny services that a family might need immediately, in order to collect data that will have general value but not necessarily value for that particular family.

Another difficulty with program evaluation research is that it is often conducted for the purposes of a particular organization or as evidence of proper use of funding for government overseers. It does not always get published in refereed journals. A number of program evaluation studies have been conducted with CCPT and FT, and these have produced very positive results (VanFleet, 1983, 1991). Indeed, the results were sufficient to convince key decision makers to continue to fund the programs.

Qualitative research has a different purpose and methodology from those of quantitative research, and therefore it offers a different type of information. Qualitative studies often involve unobtrusive observation, participant observation, and ethological methods. When done correctly, they also involve specific data evaluation methods that suggest future lines of inquiry. Qualitative studies are valuable for developing theory in new fields of interest, as well as for providing tentative explanations for the results obtained in quantitative studies. For example, if a quantitative study shows that play therapy is effective, a qualitative inquiry might contribute to the understanding of "why." Some of the quantitative studies done to date have included some qualitative components, although a search of the literature has not yielded a full qualitative study done on CCPT or FT. Even so, the qualitative aspects of existing studies have suggested hypotheses about the nature of CCPT and FT in clinical practice that warrant further testing. In addition, there are a substantial number of clinicians who, as parents, participated in nondirective play sessions with their own children as part of their preparation to FT. No known study of their experiences has been conducted, but their informal comments have attested to the power of the approach. In many cases, such clinician-parents have told us that their own experiences with family play sessions were so positive that they sought further training and supervision in FT.

In summary, many types of studies can inform practitioners about therapeutic modalities that work best with their child and family clients. The use of CCPT and FT has increased dramatically through recent decades, and surveys and program evaluation studies have pointed to their potential value. Even the quantity of research has increased substantially with time (Bratton et al., 2005; VanFleet et al., 2005). Well-designed and executed quantitative research that is properly interpreted within its limitations provides the most solid platform upon which clinicians can base their work. Well-done qualitative research can generate new questions for study and provide more details about how and why the therapy works as it does. In essence, quantitative research builds the foundation and frame of the "house," while qualitative studies offer the "décor." The next section summarizes the current state of empirical support for CCPT and FT.

Summary of Empirical Support for CCPT and FT

There is considerable evidence that both CCPT and FT are effective. In this section, we first describe four key references for play therapy and FT research, and we then summarize the research results. These four resources provide information from the most controlled quantitative studies completed on play therapy in general, CCPT in particular, and FT.

Four Key Resources

• Bratton, S. C., Ray, D., Rhine, T., & Jones, L. (2005). The efficacy of play therapy with children: A meta-analytic review of treatment outcomes. *Professional Psychology: Research and Practice*, 36(4), 376–390. This article represents the largest meta-analysis of play therapy research outcomes to date. A meta-analysis allows researchers to compensate for the small sample sizes prevalent in much therapy research by combining the outcomes of many studies into an overall treatment effect. In this important meta-analysis, the authors found 93 studies that met their strict criteria for inclusion. The meta-analysis examined 74 studies of nondirective/humanistic play therapy, including 26 studies of FT, that used control or comparison groups. The article clearly defines the criteria used, the rationale for various decisions, the results, and a helpful discussion of what conclusions can and cannot be drawn from this project. The efficacy of play therapy and FT was demonstrated definitively.

• **Ray, D. (2006). Evidence-based play therapy. In C. E. Schaefer & H. G. Kaduson (Eds.),** Contemporary play therapy: Theory, research, and practice (pp. 136–157). New York: Guilford Press. This chapter outlines the importance, history, and outcomes of play therapy research. It includes clear descriptions of research dilemmas and shortcomings—especially in regard to studies done with actual clients in real-world venues, such as schools, hospitals, independent practice settings, and clinics. It highlights a sampling of studies that demonstrate the robustness of play therapy, with a focus on CCPT. It provides information useful to clinicians who wish to conduct research, as well as to end users who might wish to demonstrate to referral sources, funding organizations, or administrators that play therapy is evidence-based.

• **Reddy, L., Files-Hall, T., & Schaefer, C. (Eds.). (2005).** Empirically based play interventions for children. Washington, DC: American Psychological Association. This book's chapters summarize the research on different types or applications of play therapy. The volume is a comprehensive resource that demonstrates the empirical bases of play therapy interventions with a wide range of problems.

• **VanFleet, R., Ryan, S., & Smith, S. (2005). Filial Therapy: A critical review. In L. Reddy, T. Files-Hall, & C. Schaefer (Eds.),** Empirically based play interventions for children (pp. 241–264). Washington, DC: American Psychological Association. This chapter of the Reddy et al. book summarizes the historical research on FT, in which one of us (Sywulak) played a seminal role. It then highlights some of the best-controlled more recent studies of FT, illustrating its power in helping families with many different problems and circumstances. It closes with recommendations for clinicians who wish to contribute to the ongoing development of empirical evidence for the effectiveness of FT. The chapter highlights the reasons why FT is presently considered the most empirically supported form of play therapy.

Findings

The meta-analysis of play therapy research by Bratton et al. (2005) is the most comprehensive to date. As noted above, they examined 93 studies that met their criteria as having defined the use of play therapy, a control or comparison group with pre- and posttesting, and sufficient data for effect sizes to be calculated. These studies represented a wide range of presenting problems and a total of 3,248 children. Bratton et al. examined both published and unpublished studies, in order to reduce publication bias (studies are more likely to be published if they have statistically significant results). The meta-analysis yielded an overall effect size of 0.80. This is considered a large effect size, meaning that children receiving play therapy performed 0.80 standard deviations above children who did not receive play therapy. This study and its detailed analyses clearly showed that play therapy is effective with a broad spectrum of problems, and it was equally effective for children with internalizing, externalizing, and combined presenting issues.

The study authors also explored a number of treatment characteristics, including the type of play therapy or its theoretical basis as either nondirective (CCPT, humanistic) or directive. The mean effect size for the 73 studies falling into the nondirective category was 0.92. This result clearly attests to the effectiveness of CCPT approaches. Other analyses demonstrated that effectiveness was maintained regardless of setting, child gender and age, and presenting problems.

Bratton et al. (2005) also examined studies in terms of individuals delivering the play interventions. They separated FT studies in which trained parents conducted play sessions with their own children under the supervision of a mental health professional. These 22 studies yielded a very high effect size of 1.15, whereas the effect size for play therapy offered directly by a mental health professional was 0.72. This is strong evidence that parent involvement in FT offers a substantial bonus in terms of outcomes.

In summary, the meta-analysis showed that play therapy is effective, that nondirective play therapy is very effective, and that the inclusion of parents in FT is highly effective. Although any meta-analysis is limited by the quality of studies included in it, the Bratton et al. research is a major step forward in demonstrating the empirical evidence for the value of play therapy as an intervention for children and families.

Other resources have compiled and analyzed the research to date relating to play therapy, and more specifically to CCPT and FT. The Reddy et al. (2005) book explores evidence for a wide range of play therapy modalities and a diverse set of problems or circumstances. This volume clearly demonstrates the empirical basis of play therapy and recommends future directions for inquiry. Ray (2006) outlines several controlled studies that used CCPT or a nondirective play therapy group as the treatment, all of which show the applicability and power of these methods. She also offers a clear and important discussion of the current state of play therapy research, including implications for future studies. VanFleet et al. (2005) have done much the same with FT studies, providing a summary of the historical research on this combined family therapy–play therapy approach, and discussing 10 recent controlled studies. This description shows the effectiveness and the robustness of FT with different problems, settings, and cultures. This chapter also highlights ways that clinicians can add to the evidence base of FT.

In summary, there are many sources of information about the effectiveness of CCPT and FT, ranging from clinicians' self-reports, case studies, and surveys through the more rigorous and definitive controlled research studies. Although more outcome and process research is needed, the empirical support for these methods is strong. Readers are encouraged to obtain the four references described here, to gain a deeper depth of understanding of the evidence to date. This material is encouraging for those who wish to employ play therapy with their child and family clients, and who wish to demonstrate CCPT and FT as empirically supported approaches.

CHAPTER 14

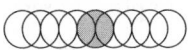

Developing Competence
in Child-Centered Play Therapy

CCPT is deceptively simple. One might be tempted to think that learning four skills and a bit about interpreting children's play would be quickly accomplished. In fact, however, there are many subtleties and nuances to the effective practice of CCPT. To become proficient in its use, therapists must receive training followed by supervised practice. This chapter details the types of training that should be considered, factors to consider in selecting a CCPT supervisor or case consultant, other resources that may be useful, and CCPT and play therapy credentials that can be obtained.

Training

As the field of play therapy continues to grow, increasing numbers of university programs are offering courses in play therapy. Some of these courses are introductory in nature, whereas others offer substantial depth in the practice of play therapy, including CCPT. For professionals who have already completed their graduate programs, various workshops and intensive training programs in play therapy and CCPT are available.

The vast array of play therapy conferences and training programs now offered in the United States and abroad can be overwhelming. Where does one start? Because CCPT is so widely practiced, is increasingly in demand, and is foundational in many ways to other forms of play therapy, it is a good place to start. CCPT training shows therapists some of the most effective ways to build rapport and attend to children's developmental and psychosocial needs, and this knowledge can be transferred to most other forms of play therapy and child therapy.

In selecting a training program, there are several things to consider. A training program about "play therapy" is not necessarily about CCPT, and the description should reveal the scope and depth of the training. In the United States, the type of nondirective play therapy inspired by the work of Rogers and Axline is frequently called CCPT, as we have done in this volume. In the United Kingdom, it is more often called "nondirective play therapy." Other names have been applied, such as "person-centered play therapy" or "client-centered play therapy," but to avoid confusion, it is best to determine whether the training follows Axline's eight principles.

Because there are different interpretations of these eight principles, there are different styles of conducting CCPT, as we have noted earlier. When therapists are considering a training program, it is advisable for them to ask for details about the stylistic interpretations that are represented within it. These differences do not suggest a single correct way to conduct CCPT, as there is no such thing, but the content of some training programs may differ from the content of this volume as a result of these varying interpretations of Axline's work. Even so, despite some variations in style or in the implementation of some skills, there tends to be considerable agreement among different professionals and programs offering CCPT training. In this volume, we have tried to articulate our reasons for conducting the therapy as we do. When therapists encounter a different method or interpretation of some aspects of CCPT, it can be valuable to ask the instructors or supervisors to share their own reasons for doing things as they do. It is part of the journey toward becoming an effective practitioner of CCPT to consider these points and arrive at one's own conclusions about how Axline's eight principles apply to one's own work.

Introductions to CCPT are available at conference presentations, as part of a broader play therapy curriculum at universities, through 1-day or 2-day introductory workshops, and through books and DVD programs. These provide good opportunities to learn the basic premises and practices of CCPT, but they are not sufficient for mastery of the attitudes and skills needed for proficiency. Many people have developed misunderstandings about CCPT by attending only a short program that offers a few video clips of play sessions, without providing the contextual backdrop for the process. Further training is absolutely necessary.

Graduate courses that devote *at least* half a semester to CCPT, intensive workshops lasting 3 or 4 days for a small number of people, or small sequential workshops that offer increasingly advanced training are needed to help professionals develop their CCPT abilities properly. The best training involves actual practice of CCPT skills through either role plays and/or actual work with children, after which the instructor provides individualized feedback to each participant. An instructor's observation of and feedback about each individual's skills during practice sessions optimizes the learning experience for CCPT. Large groups using only small breakout groups for practice do not supply this individualized feedback, although they may be helpful at the introductory level.

Beyond these trainings, it is advisable for therapists to obtain supervised practice of their use of CCPT with actual children. This is covered in more depth in the next section. Advanced CCPT courses help hone therapists' understanding and use of CCPT in a variety of settings with a range of problems and with more complex cases.

Supervision

As with most forms of therapy, training represents only the first important steps toward mastery. Many therapists learn much more from actual experience applying what they have learned in the training. In our experiences of training and supervising thousands of CCPT therapists, the most competent therapists are those who receive supervision from experienced CCPT practitioners and supervisors.

Selecting the right supervisor for CCPT work is important. Although it is advisable to learn from a Registered Play Therapist-

Supervisor (see *www.a4pt.org*) or someone with an equivalent credential in play therapy in general, it is also essential that the supervisor have substantial training and experience with CCPT specifically. Potential supervisors should be willing to share their own history of training and supervised practice: where they obtained their CCPT training, from whom they received supervision, and how long they have been using CCPT. Because the practice of CCPT is becoming so widespread—it is increasingly being used around the world—there are many qualified supervisors available. Supervisors have a large impact on professionals' eventual competence and confidence in using particular methods of therapy, so it is well worth the time and effort to find one who is highly experienced and qualified.

Sometimes a supervisor will have a somewhat different stylistic approach to the conduct of CCPT from the one a therapist has learned in training. When such differences are discovered, it is important that the two professionals discuss them until a point of mutual satisfaction is reached. Learning to become an effective play therapist is a process that needs to be embedded in a dynamic and respectful supervisory relationship. There is no room for dogma, which limits the exploration and professional development that comes from experience and supervisory feedback. No two play therapists are exactly alike. Supervisors should be able to explain why they are making the recommendations that they do; supervisees need to be open to this input, interested in sharing and exploring their own reactions about the sessions, willing to try to improve their skills, and eager to take an active part in their own learning process.

Supervision can take many forms: in person; by using videos; via telephone or e-mail; and/or by using a webcam system. Most would agree that live supervision is far preferable to other forms, but sometimes it is not feasible, especially in rural areas or countries where no CCPT supervisors are nearby. Phone and e-mail supervision can sometimes be combined, but great care must be taken to ensure confidentiality, as these avenues are not always completely private. Whether the supervision is done in person or from a distance, the use of video adds tremendously to the quality of the process. To gain maximum benefit from supervision, therapists are urged to submit videos of their CCPT sessions at least some of the time. This permits supervisors to see and hear subtleties that might go unrecognized when sessions are simply discussed without the use of video.

Resources Available

Several resources that augment or extend the material covered in this volume are available. These are listed below with brief descriptions.

Live Workshops

Live workshops in CCPT are available through numerous sources (too many to list here). All three of us offer introductory, intermediate, and advanced training programs in CCPT in the United States and abroad, and we can be contacted as noted below. One of us (VanFleet) can make referrals to reputable, qualified trainers in various locations throughout the world.

- **Risë VanFleet, PhD, RPT-S**
  Family Enhancement and Play Therapy Center, Inc.
  P.O. Box 613, Boiling Springs, PA 17007
  Phone: 717-249-4707
  Website: *www.play-therapy.com*
  e-mail: *Risevanfleet@aol.com*

- **Andrea E. Sywulak, PhD, RPT-S**
  Sywulak and Weiss Psychological Associates, LLC
  928 Jaymor Road, Suite A-120, Southampton, PA 18966
  Phone: 215-355-8812
  e-mail: *asywulakPC@gmail.com*

- **Cynthia Caparosa Sniscak, LPC, RPT-S**
  Beech Street Program, LLC
  20-A Beech Street, Carlisle, PA 17013
  Phone: 717-245-2404
  Website: *www.beechstreetprogram.com*
  e-mail: *csnis@yahoo.com*

DVD Workshop

Available from *www.play-therapy.com* (see this site for a listing of its contents), the following DVD workshop covers many details of CCPT and illustrates them with an actual CCPT session. It consists of a 3-hour DVD set and accompanying handout manual.

- VanFleet, R. (2006). *Child-Centered Play Therapy: A DVD Workshop*. Boiling Springs, PA: Play Therapy Press.

Credentials

Most of the credentials currently available are for play therapy in general or for FT. Readers are invited to visit the "Links" page of *www.play-therapy.com* to learn more about associations for play therapy professionals in a number of different countries. Efforts are made to keep this page current.

Credentials available for the Guerney-inspired form of CCPT covered in this book are available from the following organizations, which also offer credentials for FT.

- **Family Enhancement and Play Therapy Center, Inc.**
  Phone: 717-249-4707
  Website: *www.play-therapy.com*

- **National Institute of Relationship Enhancement**
  Phone: 301-986-1479
  Website: *www.nire.org*

Conclusion

CCPT is an empirically supported method of play therapy that has been used successfully for a wide range of child problems. Many therapists using CCPT for the first time with their clients use the word "magic" to describe the results. Although children's responses to this approach do indeed seem magical at times, this is perhaps attributable to the special qualities of childhood. Spontaneity, imagination, and playfulness are characteristics that adults sometimes leave behind in their busy, stressful lives. This is unfortunate, because these are the very features that support stress reduction, creativity, healthy relationships, and well-being. CCPT is unique because it opens the door for children to be who they are. When adults offer empathy, unconditional positive regard, and genuineness, they enter once again the very special world of childhood. The ability to help distressed children and their families live their lives with greater happiness and richness is its own reward.

References

Adalist-Estrin, A. (1986). Parenting from behind bars. *Family Resource Coalition— FRC Report, 1,* 12–13.

Allan, J. A. B. (2008). *Inscapes of the child's world: Jungian counseling in schools and clinics.* New York: Continuum.

American Psychiatric Association. (2000). *Diagnostic and statistical manual of mental disorders* (4th ed., text rev.). Washington, DC: Author.

Axline, V. M. (1947). *Play therapy.* Boston: Houghton Mifflin.

Axline, V. M. (1964). *Dibs: In search of self.* New York: Ballantine Books.

Axline, V. M. (1969). *Play therapy* (rev. ed.). New York: Ballantine Books.

Barabash, K. J. (2004). Developmental filial therapy: Process–outcome research on strengthening child–parent relationships through play in a setting for victims of domestic violence (Doctoral dissertation, University of Victoria, Victoria, British Columbia). *Dissertation Abstracts International, 64*(7), 3513B.

Bekoff, M., & Byers, J. A. (Eds.). (1998). *Animal play: Evolutionary, comparative, and ecological perspectives.* Cambridge, UK: Cambridge University Press.

Benedict, H. E. (2006). Object relations play therapy: Applications to attachment problems and relational trauma. In C. E. Schaefer & H. G. Kaduson (Eds.), *Contemporary play therapy: Theory, research, and practice* (pp. 3–27). New York: Guilford Press.

Bergen, D. (2009). Play as the learning medium for future scientists, mathematicians, and engineers. *American Journal of Play, 1*(4), 413–428.

Bernstein, N. (2001). *The lost children of Wilder: The epic struggle to change foster care.* New York: Vintage Books.

Bratton, S. C., Ray, D., Rhine, T., & Jones, L. (2005). The efficacy of play therapy with children: A meta-analytic review of treatment outcomes. *Professional Psychology: Research and Practice, 36*(4), 376–390.

Bronfenbrenner, U. (1979). *The ecology of human development.* Cambridge, MA: Harvard University Press.

Brown, S., & Vaughan, C. (2009). *Play: How it shapes the brain, opens the imagination, and invigorates the soul.* New York: Avery.

Burghardt, G. M. (2005). *The genesis of animal play: Testing the limits.* Cambridge, MA: The MIT Press.

Caplin, W., & Pernet, K. (in press). *Group filial therapy for at-risk families: A leader's manual for an effective short-term model.* Boiling Springs, PA: Play Therapy Press.

Chudacoff, H. P. (2007). *Children at play.* New York: New York University Press.

Clark, C. D., & Miller, P. J. (1998). Play. In H. Friedman (Ed.), *Encyclopedia of mental health* (Vol. 3, pp. 189–197). San Diego, CA: Academic Press.

Cochran, N., Nordling, W., & Cochran, J. (2010). *Child centered play therapy: A practical guide to developing therapeutic relationships with children.* Hoboken, NJ: Wiley.

Cohen, L. J. (2001). *Playful parenting.* New York: Ballantine Books.

Drewes, A. (Ed.). (2009). *Blending play therapy with cognitive behavioral therapy: Evidence-based and other effective treatments and techniques.* Hoboken, NJ: Wiley.

Ekman, P. (2007). *Emotions revealed* (2nd ed.). New York: Holt Paperbacks.

Elkind, D. (2007). *The power of play.* Cambridge, MA: Da Capo Lifelong Books.

Ellis, C. M., & Carlson, J. (2009). *Cross cultural awareness and social justice in counseling.* New York: Taylor & Francis.

Else, P. (2009). *The value of play.* New York: Continuum.

Fagen, R. (1981). *Animal play behavior.* New York: Oxford University Press.

Freud, A. (1974). The methods of child analysis. In *The writings of Anna Freud.* New York: International Universities Press. (Original work published 1927)

Gallo-Lopez, L. (2001). TV show storyboard. In H. G. Kaduson & C. E. Schaefer (Eds.), *101 more favorite play therapy techniques* (pp. 8–10). Northvale, NJ: Jason Aronson.

Gallo-Lopez, L., & Schaefer, C. E. (Eds.). (2005). *Play therapy with adolescents* (2nd ed.). Lanham, MD: Aronson.

Gil, E., & Drewes, A. A. (Eds.). (2005). *Cultural issues in play therapy.* New York: Guilford Press.

Ginsberg, B. G. (1976). Parents as therapeutic agents: The usefulness of filial therapy in a community mental health center. *American Journal of Community Psychology, 4*(1), 47–54.

Ginsberg, B. G. (1997). *Relationship enhancement family therapy.* New York: Wiley.

Ginsberg, B. G. (2003). An integrated, holistic model of child-centered family therapy. In R. VanFleet & L. F. Guerney (Eds.), *Casebook of filial therapy* (pp. 21–47). Boiling Springs, PA: Play Therapy Press.

Ginsberg, B. G., Sywulak, A. E., & Cramer, T. A. (1984). Beyond behavior modification: Client-centered play therapy with the retarded. *Academic Psychology Bulletin, 6*(1), 321–334.

Ginsburg, K. R. (2007). The importance of play in promoting healthy child development and maintaining strong parent–child bonds. *Pediatrics, 119*(1), 182–191.

Guerney, B. G., Jr. (1964). Filial therapy: Description and rationale. *Journal of Consulting Psychology, 28*(4), 303–310.

Guerney, B. G., Jr. (Ed.). (1969). *Psychotherapeutic agents: New roles for non-professionals, parents, and teachers.* New York: Holt, Rinehart & Winston.

Guerney, B. G., Jr., & Flumen, A. B. (1970). Teachers as psychotherapeutic agents for withdrawn children. *Journal of Psychology, 8*(2), 107–113.

Guerney, B. G., Jr., & Guerney, L. F. (1961). Analysis of interpersonal relationships as an aid to understanding family dynamics. A case report. *Journal of Clinical Psychology, 17*(3), 225–228.

Guerney, B. G., Stollak, G., & Guerney, L. F. (1970). A format for a new mode of psychological practice: Or, how to escape a zombie. *Consulting Psychologist, 2*(2), 97–105.

Guerney, B. G., Jr., Stollak, G., & Guerney, L. F. (1971). The practicing psychologist as educator: An alternative to the medical practitioner model. *The Counseling Psychologist, 2*(3), 276–282.

Guerney, B. G., Jr., & Stover, L. (1971). *Filial therapy: Final report on MH 1826401.* (Available from the National Institute of Relationship Enhancement, 12500 Blake Road, Silver Spring, MD 20904)

Guerney, L. F. (1976). Filial therapy program. In D. H. Olsen (Ed.), *Treating relationships* (pp. 67–91). Lake Mills, IA: Graphic.

Guerney, L. F. (1983). Introduction to filial therapy: Training parents as therapists. In P. A. Keller & L. G. Ritt (Eds.), *Innovations in clinical practice: A source book* (Vol. 2, pp. 26–39). Sarasota, FL: Professional Resource Exchange.

Guerney, L. F. (1991). Parents as partners in treating behavior problems in early childhood settings. *Topics in Early Childhood Special Education, 11*(2), 74–90.

Guerney, L. F. (1995). *Parenting: A skills training manual* (5th ed.). North Bethesda, MD: IDEALS.

Guerney, L. F. (2001). Child-centered play therapy. *International Journal of Play Therapy, 10*(2), 13–31.

Guerney, L. F., & Guerney, B. G., Jr. (1987). Integrating child and family therapy. *Psychotherapy, 24*(3), 609–614.

Harris, Z. (2003). Filial therapy with incarcerated mothers in a county jail. In R. VanFleet & L. F. Guerney (Eds.), *Casebook of filial therapy* (pp. 373–384). Boiling Springs, PA: Play Therapy Press.

Hirsh-Pasek, K., Golinkoff, R. M., & Eyer, D. (2003). *Einstein never used flash cards: How our children really learn—and why they need to play more and memorize less.* New York: MJF Books.

Honoré, C. (2008). *Under pressure: Rescuing our children from the culture of hyperparenting.* New York: HarperOne.

Jernberg, A. M., & Booth, P. B. (1999). *Theraplay: Helping parents and children build better relationships through attachment based play* (2nd ed.). San Francisco: Jossey-Bass.

Jones, G. (2002). *Killing monsters: Why children need fantasy, super heroes, and make-believe violence.* New York: Basic Books.

Kaduson, H. G. (2006). *Play therapy for children with ADHD* [DVD]. Monroe Township, NJ: Author.

Knell, S. M. (1993). *Cognitive-behavioral play therapy.* Northvale, NJ: Aronson.

Kottman, T. (2002). *Partners in play: An Adlerian approach to play therapy.* Alexandria, VA: American Counseling Association.

Kottman, T., Ashby, J. S., & Degraaf, D. G. (2001). *Adventures in guidance: How to integrate fun into your guidance program.* Alexandria, VA: American Counseling Association.

Labovitz-Boik, B., & Goodwin, E. A. (2000). *Sandplay therapy: A step-by-step manual for psychotherapists of diverse orientations.* New York: Norton.

Landreth, G. L. (2002). *Play therapy: The art of the relationship* (2nd ed.). New York: Brunner-Routledge.

Landreth, G. L., & Bratton, S. C. (2006). *Child Parent Relationship Therapy (CPRT)*. New York: Routledge.

Landreth, G. L., & Lobaugh, A. (1998). Filial therapy with incarcerated fathers: Effects on parental acceptance of child, parental stress, and child adjustment. *Journal of Counseling and Development, 76,* 157–165.

Levy, D. (1938). Release therapy in young children. *Psychiatry, 1,* 387–389.

Lobaugh, A. (2003). Filial therapy with incarcerated fathers in a federal prison. In R. VanFleet & L. F. Guerney (Eds.), *Casebook of filial therapy* (pp. 373–384). Boiling Springs, PA: Play Therapy Press.

London, K. B., & McConnell, P. B. (2008). *Play together, stay together: Happy and healthy play between people and dogs*. Black Earth, WI: McConnell.

Lowenfeld, M. (1979). *The world technique*. London: Allen & Unwin.

Mandelbaum, D., & Carter, L. (2003). Filial therapy in independent practice. In R. VanFleet & L. F. Guerney (Eds.), *Casebook of filial therapy* (pp. 361–372). Boiling Springs, PA: Play Therapy Press.

McConnell, P. B. (2006). *For the love of a dog: The biology of emotion in two species* [DVD]. Meridian, ID: Tawzer Dog Videos.

Mechling, J. (2008). Gun play. *American Journal of Play, 1*(2), 192–209.

Miller, P. (2008). *Play with your dog*. Wenatchee, WA: Dogwise.

Minuchin, S. (1974). *Families and family therapy*. Cambridge, MA: Harvard University Press.

Munns, E. (Ed.). (2000). *Theraplay: Innovations in attachment-enhancing play therapy*. Northvale, NJ: Aronson.

Munns, E. (Ed.). (2009). *Applications of family and group Theraplay*. Lanham, MD: Aronson.

Nordling, W. J., & Guerney, L. F. (1999). Typical stages in the child-centered play therapy process. *Journal for the Professional Counselor, 14*(1), 17–23.

O'Connor, K. J. (2000). *The play therapy primer* (2nd ed.). New York: Wiley.

O'Connor, K. J., & Braverman, L. D. (Eds.). (2009). *Play therapy theory and practice: Comparing theories and techniques* (2nd ed.). Hoboken, NJ: Wiley.

Paley, V. G. (2004). *A child's work: The importance of fantasy play*. Chicago: University of Chicago Press.

Panksepp, J. (2005). *Affective neuroscience: The foundations of human and animal emotions*. New York: Oxford University Press.

Pellegrini, A. D. (2008). The recess debate: A disjuncture between educational policy and scientific research. *American Journal of Play, 1*(2), 181–191.

Pellegrini, A. D., & Smith, P. K. (Eds.). (2005). *The nature of play: Great apes and humans*. New York: Guilford Press.

Perry, J. P., & Branum, L. (2009). "Sometimes I pounce on twigs because I'm a meat eater": Supporting physically active play and outdoor learning. *American Journal of Play, 2*(2), 195–214.

Ramos, A. M. (2003). Filial therapy after domestic violence. In R. VanFleet & L. Guerney (Eds.), *Casebook of filial therapy* (pp. 171–183). Boiling Springs, PA: Play Therapy Press.

Ray, D. (2006). Evidence-based play therapy. In C. E. Schaefer & H. G. Kaduson (Eds.), *Contemporary play therapy: Theory, research, and practice* (pp. 136–157). New York: Guilford Press.

Reddy, L., Files-Hall, T., & Schaefer, C. (Eds.). (2005). *Empirically based play interventions for children*. Washington, DC: American Psychological Association.

Reissman, F. (1965). The "helper" therapy principle. *Social Work, 10*(2), 27–32.

Reynolds, C. A. (2003). Filial therapy with parents earning GEDs. In R. VanFleet & L. Guerney (Eds.), *Casebook of filial therapy* (pp. 351–360). Boiling Springs, PA: Play Therapy Press.

Rogers, C. R. (1951). *Client-centered therapy*. Boston: Houghton Mifflin.

Sensue, M. E. (1981). *Filial therapy follow-up study: Effects on parental acceptance and child adjustment*. Unpublished doctoral dissertation, The Pennsylvania State University, University Park, PA.

Sori, C. F. (Ed.). (2006). *Engaging children in family therapy: Creative approaches to integrating theory and research in clinical practice*. New York: Routledge.

Stanley, J. C., & Campbell, D. T. (1973). *Experimental and quasi-experimental designs for research* (10th ed.). Chicago: Rand McNally College Publishing.

Sutton-Smith, B. (1997). *The ambiguity of play*. Cambridge, MA: Harvard University Press.

Sutton-Smith, B. (2008, January–February). To play or not to play. *The Pennsylvania Gazette*, pp. 18–19.

Sweeney, D. S., & Homeyer, L. E. (1999). *The handbook of group play therapy*. San Francisco: Jossey-Bass.

Sywulak, A. E. (1978). The effect of filial therapy on parental acceptance and child adjustment (Doctoral dissertation, Pennsylvania State University, 1977). *Dissertation Abstracts International, 38*(12), 6180B.

Sywulak, A. E. (2003). If the child is the boss, the boss needs to be fired: Filial therapy for children with ODD. In R. VanFleet & L. F. Guerney (Eds.), *Casebook of filial therapy* (pp. 49–64). Boiling Springs, PA: Play Therapy Press.

Terr, L. (1990). *Too scared to cry: How trauma affects children . . . and ultimately us all*. New York: Basic Books.

VanFleet, R. (1983). *Report on the skills-training program for parents of pediatric cardiology patients*. Technical report presented to Geisinger Medical Center, Danville, PA.

VanFleet, R. (1986). Mothers' perceptions of their families' needs when one of their children has diabetes mellitus: A developmental perspective (Doctoral dissertation, Pennsylvania State University, University Park, PA, 1985). *Dissertation Abstracts International, 47*(1), 324A.

VanFleet, R. (1990). *Therapist and child responses in child-centered play therapy: A training evaluation*. Technical report presented to the Pennsylvania State Office of Mental Health, Harrisburg.

VanFleet, R. (1991). *An evaluation of the effectiveness of a home-based program combining play therapy, filial therapy, and children's intensive case management*. Technical report presented to the Pennsylvania State Office of Mental Health, Harrisburg.

VanFleet, R. (2000a). Short-term play therapy for families with chronic illness. In H. G. Kaduson & C. E. Schaefer (Eds.), *Short-term play therapy for children* (pp. 175–193). New York: Guilford Press.

VanFleet, R. (2000b). Understanding and overcoming parent resistance to play therapy. *International Journal of Play Therapy, 9*(1), 35–46.

VanFleet, R. (2004). *It's only natural: Exploring the play in play therapy workshop manual*. Boiling Springs, PA: Play Therapy Press.

VanFleet, R. (2005). *Filial therapy: Strengthening parent–child relationships through play* (2nd ed.). Sarasota, FL: Professional Resource Press.

VanFleet, R. (2006a). *Child-centered play therapy: A DVD workshop* [DVD]. Boiling Springs, PA: Play Therapy Press.

VanFleet, R. (2006b). *Introduction to filial therapy: A DVD workshop* [DVD]. Boiling Springs, PA: Play Therapy Press.

VanFleet, R. (2006c). Short-term play therapy for adoptive families: Facilitating adjustment and attachment with filial therapy. In H. G. Kaduson & C. E. Schaefer (Eds.), *Short-term play therapy for children* (2nd ed., pp. 145–168). New York: Guilford Press.

VanFleet, R. (2007). *Overcoming resistance: Engaging parents in play therapy* [DVD]. Boiling Springs, PA: Play Therapy Press.

VanFleet, R. (2008a). *Filial play therapy* [part of Jon Carlson's DVD series on children and adolescents]. Washington, DC: American Psychological Association.

VanFleet, R. (2008b). *Play therapy with kids & canines: Benefits for children's developmental and psychosocial health.* Sarasota, FL: Professional Resource Press.

VanFleet, R. (2009). *Group play therapy with adolescents and young adults: An experiential approach to prevention and intervention.* Boiling Springs, PA: Play Therapy Press.

VanFleet, R., & Guerney, L. F. (Eds.). (2003). *Casebook of filial therapy.* Boiling Springs, PA: Play Therapy Press.

VanFleet, R., Lilly, J. P., & Kaduson, H. G. (1999). Play therapy for children exposed to violence: Individual, family, and community interventions. *International Journal of Play Therapy, 8*(1), 27–42.

VanFleet, R., Ryan, S., & Smith, S. (2005). Filial therapy: A critical review. In L. Reddy, T. Files-Hall, & C. Schaefer (Eds.), *Empirically based play interventions for children* (pp. 241–264). Washington, DC: American Psychological Association.

VanFleet, R., & Sniscak, C. C. (2003a). Filial therapy for attachment-disrupted and disordered children. In R. VanFleet & L. F. Guerney (Eds.), *Casebook of filial therapy* (pp. 279–308). Boiling Springs, PA: Play Therapy Press.

VanFleet, R., & Sniscak, C. C. (2003b). Filial therapy for children exposed to traumatic events. In R. VanFleet & L. F. Guerney (Eds.), *Casebook of filial therapy* (pp. 113–137). Boiling Springs, PA.

VanFleet, R., & Sniscak, C. C. (in press). *Filial therapy for child trauma and attachment problems: Leader's manual for family groups.* Boiling Springs, PA: Play Therapy Press.

Wettig, H. H. G., Franke, U., & Fjordbak, B. S. (2006). Evaluating the effectiveness of Theraplay. In C. E. Schaefer & H. G. Kaduson (Eds.), *Contemporary play therapy: Theory, research, and practice* (pp. 103–135). New York: Guilford Press.

White, J., Draper, K., & Flynt, M. (2003). Kinder training: A school counselor and teacher consultation model integrating filial therapy and Adlerian theory. In R. VanFleet & L. F. Guerney (Eds.), *Casebook of filial therapy* (pp. 331–350). Boiling Springs, PA: Play Therapy Press.

Wilson, K., & Ryan, V. (2005). *Play therapy: A non-directive approach for children and adolescents* (2nd ed.). London: Ballière Tindall.

Winerman, L. (2009). Playtime in peril. *Monitor on Psychology, 40*(8), 50–52.

Wright, C., & Walker, J. (2003). Using filial therapy with Head Start families. In R. VanFleet & L. F. Guerney (Eds.), *Casebook of filial therapy* (pp. 309–330). Boiling Springs, PA: Play Therapy Press.

Index

231